MONTH OF MEALS 3
A MENU PLANNER

Published by the American Diabetes Association

Cover photo:
Dinner 20

ISBN 0-945448-24-4

TABLE OF CONTENTS

ACKNOWLEDGMENTS

This publication was created by a committee of the Council on Nutritional Science and Metabolism of the American Diabetes Association (ADA). The committee members were Robin Ann Williams, MA, RD, CDE (Editor); Lois Babione, RD; Marti Chitwood, RD, CDE; Nancy Cooper, RD; and Susan L. Thom, RD, LD, CDE. Staff members of the ADA National Center also contributed to this publication, in particular Christine B. Welch, Don Jewler, Kim Fawcett, Peter Banks, and Susan H. Lau.

The recipes in *Month of Meals 3* come from several sources. We wish to acknowledge the following:

The recipes for Marinated Cucumbers and Fresh Lemonade appear in the *AMERICAN DIABETES ASSOCIATION/THE AMERICAN DIETETIC ASSOCIATION FAMILY COOKBOOK, VOLUME I*, Copyright © 1980 by American Diabetes Association, Inc., The American Dietetic Association. Used by permission of the publisher, Prentice-Hall, Inc., Englewood Cliffs, New Jersey.

The recipes for Quick Homemade Raisin Bread, Tortilla Soup, and New England Chicken Croquettes appear in the *AMERICAN DIABETES ASSOCIATION/THE AMERICAN DIETETIC ASSOCIATION FAMILY COOKBOOK, VOLUME III*, Copyright © 1987 by American Diabetes Association, Inc., The American Dietetic Association. Used by permission of the publisher, Prentice Hall Press, New York.

The recipe for Fresh Tomato Aspic appears in the *AMERICAN DIABETES ASSOCIATION/THE AMERICAN DIETETIC ASSOCIATION FAMILY COOKBOOK, VOLUME IV*, Copyright © 1991 by American Diabetes Association, Inc., The American Dietetic Association. Used by permission of the publisher, Prentice Hall Press, New York.

The recipe for Tofu Garden Quiche appears in *MORE CALCULATED COOKING*, Copyright © 1981 by Jeanne Jones. Used by permission of the publisher, 101 Productions/Cole Group, Inc., Santa Rosa, California.

The recipe for Meatless Chili appears in *MENU FOR LIFE*, Copyright © 1987 by Joan Klun Kaye and L.E. Smith. Used by permission of the publisher, Menu for Life, Inc., Rochester, Michigan.

The following recipes were used by permission of the creators: Fiesta Rice, Chicken Ratatouille, and Mike's Veal by Mike Connor; Grilled Veggies by Debra L. Edmonds; Light and Creamy Yogurt Pie and Saucy Seafood Stir Fry by Kathy England; Squash Casserole by Cathy Marett; Frosty Grapes by Cindy McAllister; Fajita in a Pita by Deborah C. McClary; Roger's Coleslaw by Roger McCullough; Vegetable Stir Fry by Shawn McLemore; Chocolate-Flavored Syrup by Debbie Pierce; and Black Bean Dip by Judy Sharpe.

All other recipes were published in *Diabetes Forecast*, ADA's monthly magazine on living better with diabetes, or were developed by the creators of *Month of Meals 3*.

For information on ordering any of the ADA cookbooks mentioned above or joining the ADA, call the ADA National Center at 1-800-232-3472 or contact your state ADA affiliate, listed in the white pages of the phone book.

People with diabetes can eat a wide variety of foods—including packaged foods, such as frozen entrees—as long as their overall diet is well balanced. Therefore, as a convenient aid to readers who want fast yet healthy meal choices, *Month of Meals 3* includes many brand or product names. The use of selected brand names does not imply that they are the only brands in a product category suitable for people with diabetes. In addition, although every attempt possible was made to ensure that these packaged foods meet calorie restrictions of individual menus, the ADA does not endorse these products or guarantee that they are appropriate for all people with diabetes. Consumers are encouraged to read food labels carefully and to consult with a health-care professional to decide whether a food is appropriate for their meal plans.

Photo at right:
Breakfast 24

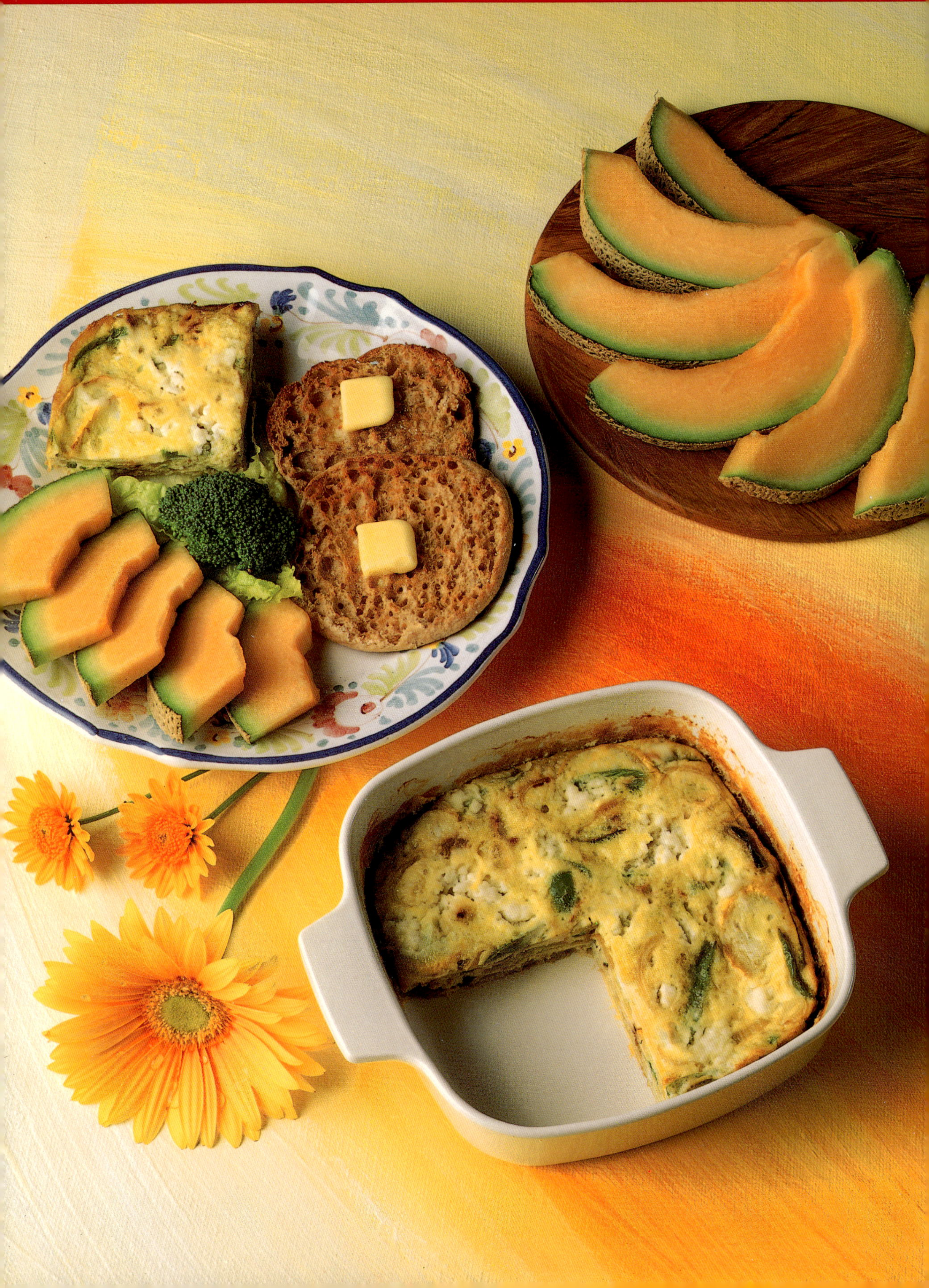

INTRODUCTION

Welcome to *Month of Meals 3*. This book is designed to help you choose healthy foods easily and quickly. There are complete menus for breakfast, lunch, dinner, and snacks. You will find many menus that can be prepared quickly, menus using convenience and fast foods for your jet-paced lifestyle, and menus emphasizing low-fat and high-fiber foods. *Month of Meals 3* is set up in a way that will allow you to mix and match meals for a month. There is also information on label reading and meal planning in times of illness.

Each day's menu—breakfast, lunch, dinner, and a snack—provides approximately 1500 calories. This figure can be adjusted up or down to meet your specific calorie requirements. A day's menus will provide about 45 to 50 percent of the calories from carbohydrate, 20 percent from protein, and about 30 percent from fat.

Month of Meals 3 allows you to choose tasty menus that meet the 1990 *Dietary Guidelines for Americans* (Dept. of Agriculture and Dept. of Health and Human Services, Home and Garden Bulletin 232).

- **Eat a variety of foods**. Eating a wide variety of different foods helps to ensure that you get all the essential vitamins, minerals, and nutrients your body needs. Variety also helps keep your interest so that your diet doesn't become boring. With *Month of Meals 3*, you don't just have one month of daily menus, you can mix and match over 19,000 combinations of breakfasts, lunches, and dinners.
- **Maintain a healthy weight**. *Month of Meals 3* allows you to add and subtract snacks to get just the right calorie intake for you to achieve and maintain a healthy body weight.
- **Choose a diet low in fat, saturated fat, and cholesterol**. *Month of Meals 3* menus average less than 300 milligrams of cholesterol per day and about 30 percent total fat. Menus emphasize choosing reduced-fat or low-fat foods. The two meals considered higher in cholesterol or saturated fat are marked for occasional use only. Refer to the section about reading labels to learn how to identify hidden fats in foods.
- **Choose a diet with plenty of vegetables, fruits, and grain products**. These foods not only add variety to your diet, but when unprocessed or unrefined, they are an important source of fiber. Unrefined foods are close in form to what Mother Nature gives us, and the closer, the better. In *Month of Meals 3*, high-fiber meals are indicated by the symbol 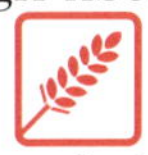
- **Use sugars only in moderation**. These recipes are low in sugar. No-sugar and low-sugar fruit spreads (jams and jellies) are recommended. Simple desserts containing limited amounts of sugar are included. Instead of sugar, you can also use artificial sweeteners that have essentially no calories, such as aspartame (Equal or NutraSweet), acesulfame-K (Sweet One or Sunette), and saccharin (Sweet 'n Low, Sugar Twin, or Sweet 10). The best artificial sweeteners to use when baking are those made of saccharin or acesulfame-K.
- **Use salt and sodium only in moderation**. Most of the menus use salt very moderately. Those menus containing higher than recommended sodium levels are noted for occasional use. Also remember that about one-third of the sodium in your diet comes from the salt shaker. The National Institutes of Health recommends a daily intake of 1,100 to 3,300 milligrams of sodium—eating three healthy meals a day will easily provide this without using the salt shaker. Gradually cut back on the salt you add at the table and in your cooking so your taste buds have time to adjust to a lower level of sodium. If sodium is reduced gradually, you will hardly notice the change.

The menus in *Month of Meals 3* have been developed using a meal planning system that divides foods into six groups: Starch/Bread, Meat and Meat Substitutes, Vegetables, Fruit, Milk, and Fat. Foods are placed into one group or another based on their nutrient make-up of carbohydrate, protein, fat, and calories.

1

Starch/Bread. This group includes whole grains (brown rice, bulgur wheat, wheat berries, oats, barley), cereal, pasta, rice, breads, starchy vegetables (potatoes, corn, lima beans), crackers, and many snack-type foods.

2

Meat and Meat Substitutes. This group includes beef, pork, lamb, veal, poultry, fish, seafood, eggs, cheese, cottage cheese, and peanut butter. The list divides these foods into lean, medium-fat, and high-fat choices.

3

Vegetables. The vegetable list is made up of nonstarchy vegetables that are either raw or cooked, such as broccoli, asparagus, green beans, cabbage, squash, carrots, salad greens, onions, and tomatoes.

4

Fruit. This list includes all varieties of fruit—fresh, frozen, canned, and dried—as well as fruit juices.

5

Milk. Included here are milk plus yogurt and buttermilk.

6

Fat. Here you find obvious fats like margarine, butter, cooking oils, mayonnaise, and salad dressings plus other high-fat foods like avocados, olives, nuts and seeds, bacon, sour cream, and cream cheese.

For a complete listing of foods and portion sizes in the six food groups, see *Exchange Lists for Meal Planning*, available from the American Diabetes Association or The American Dietetic Association or contact a registered dietitian.

Food Group	Per Serving			
	Calories	Carbohydrate (grams)	Protein (grams)	Fat (grams)
Starch/Bread	80	15	3	1
Meat and Substitutes				
Lean	55		7	3
Medium Fat	75		7	5
High Fat	100		7	8
Vegetables	25	5	2	
Fruit	60	15		
Milk				
Skim	90	12	8	1
Low Fat	120	12	8	5
Whole	150	12	8	8
Fat	45			5

USING LABELING LINGO TO YOUR ADVANTAGE

As you use *Month of Meals 3*, you will see even more familiar brand name items from the grocery store shelves than in *Month of Meals* or *Month of Meals 2*. This is because we know that you want to use convenience foods on your busy days and that it is unrealistic to expect anyone to cook from scratch every day!

A trip to the grocery store can give you information overload: there are 15,000 food products to confront in the 30 minutes or so you have for shopping. Certainly, it is an information-processing nightmare to read all the labels and sort out the healthiest foods from the rest. So, average shoppers usually just resort to buying the old familiar products they have selected in the past, giving up on attempting to interpret the plethora of new products. Adding to the confusion are the new sweeteners and low-fat products and their accompanying label claims . . . what's a health-conscious person to do?

At the start of your next trip, remember to shop the perimeter of the store first: most grocery stores are organized such that the basic four food groups make up the four enclosing walls—produce, dairy, meat, and breads. Fill your cart with these nutritious essentials first, then proceed down only the aisles necessary to complete your grocery list. And take the time to study product labels as you go. This habit will assure that you find a variety of healthy foods to meet your nutrient needs successfully each day. What follows are some guidelines to help you select specific groups of foods commonly found in the grocery store.

Lunch meat. Lean or greater than 90 percent fat-free meats should contain 30 to 35 calories and about 1 gram of fat per ounce.

Red meat. Beef, veal, and pork are usually labeled with animal name, body part, and type of cut (for instance, pork loin chops) and are graded Prime (highest in fat), Choice, or Select (lowest in fat). Choose Select grades and lean body parts, such as the loin, tenderloin, round, or leg. You can ask your butcher to preportion the servings to 4 ounces of raw meat each.

Fish. Choose fresh fish or shellfish in the delicatessen case. Look for canned fish packed in water with no added salt. Select fresh or frozen fish without batter or breading.

Poultry. The leanest cut is boneless, skinless breast meat. Removing the skin cuts the fat in half and the cholesterol by 75 percent. Turkey or chicken processed as traditional pork-based meats, such as salami, bologna, hot dogs, and bacon, are still high in fat and should only be used occasionally. Look for ground turkey breast.

Milk. Look for skim milk or 1/2% or 1% milk. Buttermilk is usually made from skim milk, but check the label.

Yogurt. Choose sugar-free yogurts, including plain or fruited nonfat yogurt or low-fat yogurt sweetened with an artificial sweetener. Artificially sweetened yogurts are often labeled "lite" and are 50 to 100 calories per serving, depending on serving size.

Cheese. Because regular cheese has 80 to 100 calories per ounce, opt for skim milk cheeses with about 5 grams of fat per ounce or less; examples include Alpine Lace cheeses and

Kraft Light Naturals, skim milk mozzarella and farmer's cheeses, and most American flavor cheeses, excluding pasteurized processed style. Nonfat ricotta cheese is also a good choice.

Cereal. Choose cereals listing "whole" grains as the first ingredient on the label. Look for cereals that have 2 or more grams of fiber and 1 gram or less of fat per serving. They should also provide less than 5 grams of sucrose or other sugars per serving.

Bread. Just as you would for cereal, choose a bread that lists whole grains as the first ingredient on the label. Remember, two slices of diet (40-calories-per-slice) bread equal one Starch/Bread exchange.

Crackers. Choose crackers made with whole grains or mostly whole grains. The best crackers have less than 2 grams of fat per serving, which is usually 5 to 12 (or 1 ounce of) crackers, depending on their size.

Fruit and fruit juice. Buy fresh fruit or freshly squeezed 100 percent fruit juice. As long as it's 100 percent (or pure) juice, it can be fresh, canned, bottled, or frozen. Beware of juice labels stating, "made with 100 percent juice"—this means the drink contains ingredients (probably sugars) *in addition to* 100 percent juice.

Jams and jellies. Choose fruit spreads, all-fruit jams, or low-sugar spreads. If you eat less than 2 teaspoons per day, you will not have to count it in your calorie total.

Margarine and oil. The first ingredient on the label should be a liquid vegetable oil. The oil should start with an "s" (soybean, safflower, sesame, or sunflower) or a "c" (corn, cottonseed, or canola). Look for margarines and oils that contain no more than 1 gram of saturated fat per serving, usually a tablespoon. Be careful to monitor your portions of "light" and "diet" margarines—you could end up using two to three times what you normally would.

Salad dressings and sour cream. Try to choose salad dressings that contain 30 calories or less per tablespoon. These are usually labeled as reduced-calorie salad dressings and can be used in 2-tablespoon servings versus the usual 1-tablespoon serving for regular salad dressings. Any oil-free salad dressing (usually 6 calories or less per tablespoon) may be used more liberally. Light sour cream substitutes still contain fat, and many are half sour cream. As long as amounts are monitored, sour cream as a fat exchange may be used (about 2 tablespoons equals a serving). If fat, cholesterol, and calories are of major concern, just use plain yogurt flavored with chives, herbs, and spices.

Rice, pasta, and whole grains. Buy brown or wild rice of any type. Choose unfilled fresh or dried pasta, preferably made with whole wheat or vegetables such as spinach, tomato, or artichoke. Most whole grains, such as bulgur wheat, wheat berries, or oat groats, contain 100 calories per 1/2 cup of cooked grain and no fat.

Frozen entrees. Look for dinner entrees that are 350 calories or less per serving. Ideally, they should get less than 30 percent of the calories from fat; this means they should provide about 3 grams of fat per 100 calories—about 10 grams of fat per serving. Choose

USING LABELING LINGO TO YOUR ADVANTAGE

entrees with less than 800 milligrams of sodium and less than 100 milligrams of cholesterol per serving.

Soup. Low salt and low fat are the keys here. Look for frozen or canned soups with less than 500 milligrams of sodium per serving, usually 1 cup, and that get less than 30 percent of the calories from fat (see below).

Cookies. Choose cookies that contain about 60 to 80 calories per ounce (10 calories or less per cookie) and that have 2 grams or less of fat per ounce.

Frozen desserts. Choose a dessert that contains no more than 3 grams of fat per 4-ounce serving. Low-fat frozen yogurt, "light" dairy desserts, and ice milk fit in this category. Look for frozen fruit juice bars that have 55 to 70 calories per bar (and do not contain cream or coconut)—this will equal one serving of fruit.

Finding low-fat foods is one of the most important things you can do for your good health. Of all your daily calories, only about 30 percent should be from fat. Here are two ways to determine whether a product meets this guideline using information given on the label. Find the number of calories per serving and the grams of fat per serving. Then multiply the grams of fat by 9 and divide by the number of calories; when you multiply by 100, you'll have the number of calories in that food supplied by fat. Or, see where your food fits into this chart of an acceptable amount of calories from fat done by serving size:

If calories are between	Fat should be *less* than
0 and 50	2 grams
50 and 100	3 grams
100 and 150	5 grams
150 and 200	7 grams
200 and 250	8 grams
250 and 300	10 grams
300 and 350	11 grams
350 and 400	13 grams
400 and 450	15 grams
450 and 500	17 grams

Hopefully, these guidelines will make you feel more comfortable reading food labels at the grocery store. You will be more likely to try new products when you have some guidelines to follow that can help you decide whether to buy a certain food.

Be sure to pay attention to the portion sizes listed on the food label by the manufacturer. All of the nutrition information on a label relates back to that portion. This is important if you are to be able to fit that food into your meal plan. Sometimes, it is not worth it if the portion is just too small.

Remember to consume a variety of foods every day to meet your nutrient requirements. This is easily done if you do not skip any of the food groups recommended in your daily meal plan.

Enjoy the flexibility and wide variety of convenience foods at your fingertips now with *Month of Meals 3*.

FAST FOODS

Several menus in *Month of Meals 3* contain items from fast food restaurants. You are probably wondering, is fast food really a healthy choice? The answer can be yes or no, depending on what you order. When eating fast food, it is possible to consume an entire day's worth of fat, salt, and calories in just one meal! The key to making healthy fast food choices is to know exactly what you are ordering. Here are some general tips to help you do just that.

- If ordering a hamburger, choose one with just a single plain meat patty instead of a double burger with cheese or sauces, especially mayonnaise-type sauces. Also, hold the cheese—it adds 100 calories a slice as well as extra fat and sodium.

- Chicken or fish may start out lower in fat than red meat, but after it is battered, breaded, and fried, it becomes even higher in calories and fat than a hamburger. Choose chicken or fish only if it is roasted, unbreaded, grilled, baked, or broiled without fat. Use mustard instead of mayonnaise, unless low-fat mayonnaise is offered.

- "Super" hot dogs with cheese have at least 7 teaspoons of fat, about 580 calories, and a lot of sodium. You're better off sticking to a single hamburger with lettuce and tomato.

- Of all the versions of roast beef, ham and cheese, and turkey sandwiches, your best choice would be regular or junior size sandwiches rather than the larger, top-of-the-line deluxe types. You can also save calories by skipping the mayonnaise and adding lettuce, tomato, onion, and mustard instead. Plain lean roast beef, French dip, turkey or chicken breast, or lean ham are probably the leanest choices in the sandwich category, as long as you hold the bacon, cheeses, and sauces. Also, choose a bun or bread over a croissant to save fat and calories.

- Pizza can be a good fast food choice and provide valuable nutrients to your diet as well. The best choice is cheese pizza topped with mushrooms, green peppers, onions, or any other vegetables; consider asking for one-third less cheese on your pizza when ordering. If you top the pizza with pepperoni, sausage, and extra cheese, you add a lot of extra fat and sodium. Add a salad with low-fat dressing to your pizza, and you'll have an even more well-rounded meal.

- To keep fat and calories down in a fast food salad, be careful with high-fat toppings like dressings, bacon, cheeses, and seeds. Load up on lettuce and vegetables at a salad bar, and go easy on the dressing, croutons, and mayonnaise/macaroni salads. Some fast food restaurants provide individual packets of salad dressing and will tell you they only have 50 calories in a half-ounce portion. But remember, the whole packet of dressing probably contains 3 to 4 ounces, so be careful how much you use, and watch the size of the packet.

- Tacos, tostados, bean burritos, soft tacos, and other nonfried items are good choices when eating in Mexican fast food restaurants. Choose chicken items over beef, and avoid beans if they are refried in lard (ask whether they are made with lard). With all items, go easy on cheese toppings and fillings, sour cream, and guacamole. Pile on extra lettuce, tomatoes, and salsa. Limit your intake of the deep-fried taco salad shell—one taco salad can have over 1,000 calories!

- Many fast food desserts are high in fat and calories, so one option is to bring a piece of fresh fruit along from home. Or satisfy your sweet tooth with low-fat frozen yogurt (only 80 calories in 1/3 cup) or a small ice milk cone. Ices, sorbets, and sherbets generally have less fat and fewer calories than ice cream but are a significant source of sugar.

- Choosing lunch or dinner at a fast food restaurant may be easier than breakfast, because breakfast items tend to be higher in fat. Try plain English muffins or toast; be aware that other kinds of muffins can be loaded with sugar. Request no butter or margarine and low-sugar jam or jelly instead. Add fruit juice or low-fat or skim milk. Several restaurants offer cold cereals, pancakes without butter, or plain scrambled eggs. To be safe, bring your own low-sugar jam and sugar-free syrup.

To help you eat right, several restaurants are offering special products lower in fat. For example, McDonald's has introduced its McLean hamburger, and Arby's has a variety of leaner "light" sandwich options. Hardee's offers several selections lower in fat, such as the grilled chicken sandwich. Wendy's also has a grilled chicken sandwich served on a multigrain bun. Burger King's BK Broiler is flame-broiled chicken served on an oat bran bun. McDonald's has added a fat-free muffin to their breakfast options, but like most fat-free baked goods, it is high in sugar and should be eaten only occasionally.

Not all so-called "healthy" choices are such a good deal, however. Kentucky Fried Chicken advertises a skinless chicken that has almost as much fat as the regular version. To be sure of what you're eating, request the nutritional information on what you have ordered. Most establishments should have it available on request.

You will no doubt find it convenient or necessary to eat fast food on occasion. When you go, these guidelines will help you make good choices. An important key is to buy small and eat only at meal times. Avoid the high-fat, high-sugar, and high-sodium foods. If your weight is a concern, pay special attention to calorie values. By asking questions and knowing the nutritional values of fast food items, you can choose foods that will be consistent with your healthy diet.

For further information on the nutrient values of fast foods, check the April 1991 issue of *Diabetes Forecast* for the article "A New Look for Fast Food" (also available as a reprint from the American Diabetes Association).

FIBER

Throughout *Month of Meals 3*, we indicated high-fiber foods with the symbol 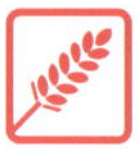

There are many reasons to eat more fiber. Studies suggest that eating a fiber-rich diet may help protect against heart disease and certain types of cancer. Also, because high-fiber foods are very filling and generally take a long time to eat, they satisfy the appetite and help with weight control. Fiber may also help to lower blood glucose levels in people with diabetes.

Fiber is the part of plant foods that we cannot digest or absorb: the roots, seeds, leaves, and outer skin. There are basically two types of fiber.

Soluble fiber dissolves in water during digestion and forms a gel in the intestinal tract. This material slows down the movement of food through the intestinal tract and can actually help delay the absorption of certain nutrients, including glucose. This is why eating soluble fiber may be of special benefit to people with diabetes.

Soluble fiber is found in oatmeal and oat bran; legumes such as dried peas, beans, and lentils; and certain fruits and vegetables, especially citrus fruits, apples, and broccoli.

Insoluble fiber doesn't dissolve in water in the intestinal tract. Instead, it retains water, swelling to several times its original size and forming a soft stool, which travels faster through the intestines. This type of fiber is most helpful in treating constipation.

Common sources of insoluble fiber are wheat bran, corn bran and popcorn, whole grains, vegetables, and nuts.

Both types of fiber are important for good nutrition, and most grains, fruits, and vegetables contain some of both types. To increase fiber in your diet, keep in mind these recommendations.

- Get half of your daily calories from high-carbohydrate foods like fruits, grains, pastas, cereals, and vegetables. Meats and dairy products do not contain dietary fiber.
- Eat a variety of fiber-rich foods. Your diet should include both soluble and insoluble fiber.
- Eat foods in their most "natural" state whenever possible: raw fruits and vegetables with their skins, whole-grain flour instead of white flour, brown rice instead of white rice, and whole fruits instead of fruit juice, for example.
- Use breads, cereals, crackers, and flour made primarily from whole grains such as whole wheat, whole oats, and any other whole grains.
- Drink plenty of water and other sugar-free fluids. Because fiber draws water into your intestinal tract, you need to drink a lot of fluids so your body can eliminate properly. (Too much fiber and not enough water can cause constipation.)
- Increase your fiber intake gradually. The sudden addition of a lot of fiber can cause intestinal gas, cramping, and diarrhea.
- It's better to get fiber from food than commercial fiber supplements. Food will give you additional nutrients besides fiber, and the long-term safety and effects of fiber supplements are not known.

HOW TO USE THIS BOOK

Month of Meals 3 allows you to choose the calorie level that best meets your needs. First, however, you need to know about how many daily calories you require. The best way to do this is to meet with a registered dietitian or certified diabetes educator who can design a meal plan with the right number of calories for your nutritional needs.

Basic Meal Plan 1500 Calories a Day

Each breakfast, each lunch, and each dinner in *Month of Meals 3* has about the same number of calories, so you can mix and match them to suit your own tastes. One day's breakfast, lunch, and dinner is about 1350 calories. By adding two 60-calorie snacks OR one 125-calorie snack, your daily total will be 1500 calories—the Basic Meal Plan. Choose any menus you like. All the portions on the menus are for one person, so you can have everything listed.

If you need more or fewer calories than the basic 1500-calorie menus provide, no problem. Adjusting meals to meet your requirements is as easy as following the instructions on the next few pages.

Basic Meal Plan Plus

If you are following a meal plan that allows you 1800 calories a day, use the chart below to adjust the Basic Meal Plan.

First, choose any menu in *Month of Meals 3* that you want. Then, move down the 1800-calorie column and follow the directions. Breakfast, lunch, and dinner are the same as in the Basic Meal Plan. The extra calories come from snacks—a 125-calorie morning snack, a 125-calorie afternoon snack, and a 170-calorie evening snack.

The chart also shows you how to reach a 2100-calorie meal plan. You may want to alter this plan to meet your needs if you are pregnant or breastfeeding.

	BASIC MEAL PLAN 1500 CALORIES	1800 CALORIES	2100 CALORIES
Breakfast	Total calories: 350	Same as Basic Meal Plan Total calories: 350	Add one meat OR one Starch/Bread to the Basic Meal Plan Total calories: 425
Morning Snack		Add one 125-calorie snack Total calories: 125	Add one 60-calorie snack Total calories: 60
Lunch	Total calories: 450	Same as Basic Meal Plan Total calories: 450	Add one Starch/Bread AND one Fat to the Basic Meal Plan Total calories: 575
Afternoon Snack		Add one 125-calorie snack Total calories: 125	Add one 125-calorie snack Total calories: 125
Dinner	Total calories: 550	Same as Basic Meal Plan Total calories: 550	Add one Starch/Bread AND one Milk to the Basic Meal Plan Total calories: 720
Evening Snack	Two 60-calorie snacks OR one 125-calorie snack Total calories: 125	Add one 170-calorie snack Total calories: 170	Add one 170-calorie snack Total calories: 170

Basic Meal Plan Minus*

If you are following a meal plan that allows you 1200 calories a day, use the chart below to adjust the Basic Meal Plan.

First, choose any menu in *Month of Meals 3* that you want. Then, move down the 1200-calorie column and follow the directions: Eliminate one starch or one milk for breakfast from the Basic Meal Plan. Eliminate one fruit at lunch from the Basic Meal Plan. Eliminate one fat at dinner from the Basic Meal Plan. There are no snacks in the 1200-calorie meal plan.

This chart shows you how to reach a 1200- and a 1350-calorie meal plan.

*To meet your body's most basic nutrient needs, you need to eat at least 1200 calories a day.

	1200 CALORIES	1350 CALORIES	BASIC MEAL PLAN 1500 CALORIES
Breakfast	Eliminate one Starch/Bread or one Milk from Basic Meal Plan Total calories: 270	Same as Basic Meal Plan Total calories: 350	Total calories: 350
Morning Snack			
Lunch	Eliminate one Fruit from Basic Meal Plan Total calories: 390	Same as Basic Meal Plan Total calories: 450	Total calories: 450
Afternoon Snack			
Dinner	Eliminate one Fat from Basic Meal Plan Total calories: 505	Same as Basic Meal Plan Total calories: 550	Total calories: 550
Evening Snack			Two 60-calorie snacks OR one 125-calorie snack Total calories: 125

Sample Meal Plan #1

Here's how to adjust the Basic Meal Plan (1500 calories) for about a 1200-calorie diet.

Meal		Calories	
Breakfast		350	
Plus or minus -1 (#) Starch/Bread (type of serving) serving(s)		-80	Subtotal 270
Lunch		450	
Plus or minus -1 (#) Fruit (type of serving) serving(s)		-60	Subtotal 390
Dinner		550	
Plus or minus -1 (#) Fat (type of serving) serving(s)		-45	Subtotal 505
	TOTAL DAILY CALORIES		1165

Sample Meal Plan #2

Here's how to adjust the Basic Meal Plan (1500 calories) for about a 2200-calorie diet.

Meal		Calories	
Breakfast		350	
Plus or minus +1 (#) Starch/Bread (type of serving) serving(s)		+80	Subtotal 430
Lunch		450	
Plus or minus +1 (#) Fruit (type of serving) serving(s)		+60	
+1 (#) Fat (type of serving) serving(s)		+45	Subtotal 555
Dinner		550	
Plus or minus + 1 (#) Starch/Bread (type of serving) serving(s)		+80	
+1 (#) Med-Fat Meat (type of serving) serving(s)		+75	
+1 (#) Fat (type of serving) serving(s)		+45	Subtotal 750
Snacks (Morning, Afternoon, and/or Evening)		125	
+2 (#) Starch/Bread (type of serving) serving(s)			
+2 (#) Milk or Meat (type of serving) serving(s)		340	Subtotal 465
	TOTAL DAILY CALORIES		2200

Your Meal Plan

Meal	Calories	
Breakfast	_______	
Plus or minus		
___ ___________ serving(s) # (type of serving)	_______	Subtotal _______
Morning Snack		
___ ___________ serving(s) # (type of serving)	_______	Subtotal _______
Lunch	_______	
Plus or minus		
___ ___________ serving(s) # (type of serving)	_______	
___ ___________ serving(s) # (type of serving)	_______	Subtotal _______
Afternoon Snack		
___ ___________ serving(s) # (type of serving)	_______	Subtotal _______
Dinner	_______	
Plus or minus		
___ ___________ serving(s) # (type of serving)	_______	
___ ___________ serving(s) # (type of serving)	_______	
___ ___________ serving(s) # (type of serving)	_______	Subtotal _______
Evening Snack		
___ ___________ serving(s) # (type of serving)	_______	Subtotal _______
	TOTAL DAILY CALORIES	_______

HOW TO USE THIS BOOK

Just as in *Month of Meals* and *Month of Meals 2*, the pages in this book are divided into thirds so that each menu (breakfast, lunch, or dinner) appears on a separate segment. You can either follow each day's meal plan in sequence or flip back and forth between the various menus for added variety.

For example, on one day you may have Breakfast 10, Lunch 2, Dinner 28, and 125-calorie Snack 8 for a total of 1500 calories.

Many of the breakfasts and lunches can be prepared quickly. Many dinners, too, are quick and easy. If you are in a hurry, the following dinners are quick choices: 6, 7, 9, 11, 14, 15, 17, 18, 23, 24, 26, and 27. Quick-choice meals are marked with the symbol 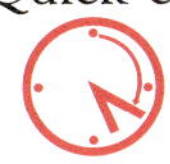 Meals made quickly with microwavable items are indicated with the symbol 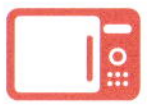

Also note that the menus high in fiber are flagged as 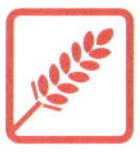 to help you make higher fiber choices.

Many recipes in this book yield more than the one serving called for in the menus. The total number of servings (yield) and the single serving size are listed at the top of each recipe.

To avoid leftovers, prepare the recipes in *Month of Meals 3* for the whole family. Then, everyone can get the benefits of eating right, and you won't feel isolated or deprived by having to eat "special" meals. Consider saving leftovers for lunches or snacks.

The recipes in this book use these standard abbreviations:

Tbsp. = tablespoon
tsp. = teaspoon
oz. = ounce
lb. = pound

Tips for Healthy Eating

You may:

- use commercial (canned, dry, or frozen) or homemade soups with these menus, but note that they are usually high in sodium, so choose reduced-fat and reduced-sodium varieties.
- use no-sugar or low-sugar fruit spreads (jams or jellies). Limit yourself to 1 to 2 teaspoons (less than 20 calories) per serving.
- use 1 tablespoon of regular salad dressing or 2 tablespoons of reduced-calorie salad dressing interchangeably. Salad dressings that contain less than 6 calories per tablespoon can be used more liberally.
- have free raw vegetables on some menus, which can include salad greens and moderate servings of carrot or celery sticks, tomatoes, cucumbers, green peppers, radishes, and the like.
- use butter-flavored granules, such as Butter Buds or Molly McButter, to season vegetables, potatoes, rice, or noodles.
- use 1/4 cup egg substitute to replace each egg in a recipe.
- add your choice of calorie-free beverages, such as coffee, hot or iced tea, mineral water, diet sodas, and sugar-free flavored seltzers.
- use skim or 1% milk in all menus and recipes.
- measure meat portions after cooking. Four ounces of uncooked meat shrinks to about 3 ounces (about the size of a deck of cards) after cooking.

Colds, flu, or dental work causing a sore mouth can change the way you usually eat. When you cannot eat your usual foods, soft or liquid replacements may be necessary. It helps to know in advance specific sick day instructions from your doctor.

Remember, you still need to follow the basic guidelines for numbers and types of exchanges for each meal (breakfast: 2 Starch/Bread, 1 Fruit, 1 Skim Milk or Meat, and 1 Fat; lunch: 2 Starch/Bread, 2 Meat or Milk, 0-1 Vegetable, 1 Fruit, and 1 Fat; dinner: 2 Starch/Bread, 2-3 Meat or Milk, 1-2 Vegetable, 1 Fruit, and 2 Fat). If you cannot tolerate meats, try the Milk exchange foods instead. If you have diabetes, you may want to spread the contents of a liquid meal over two to four hours to avoid a rapid rise in blood glucose.

Here are sample menus to use when a diet of nonsolid foods or soft, easily digested foods is required. Each meal supplies the same calories as the other breakfasts, lunches, or dinners in this book but may contain more carbohydrates.

	Liquid Menus	Soft Menus
Breakfast	1 cup oatmeal 1/2 cup orange juice 1 cup low-fat milk	1 soft scrambled egg or 1/4 cup egg substitute 2 slices bread or toast 1 Tbsp. reduced-calorie margarine 2 tsp. low-sugar fruit spread 1/2 cup applesauce
Lunch	1 cup cream of chicken soup 1/2 cup low-fat ice cream 1/2 cup tomato juice 1/2 cup apple juice	1/2 cup cottage cheese 6 saltines 6 vanilla wafers 2 canned low-sugar peach halves
Dinner	1 cup Nabisco Cream of Wheat 1 cup low-fat milk 1/2 cup sugar-free banana pudding 1/2 cup tomato juice 1/2 cup orange juice	3 oz. baked chicken 1/2 cup mashed potatoes 1/2 cup cooked carrots 1/2 cup green beans 1/2 cup applesauce 1 slice of bread 2 tsp. margarine

Substitutions

1 serving of Starch/Bread:
- 1/4 cup sherbet
- 1/2 cup pasta
- 1/2 cup mashed potatoes
- 3 graham cracker squares
- 3/4 to 1 cup soup with rice or noodles
- 1 slice bread
- 1/2 cup cooked cereal
- 1/3 cup rice
- 6 saltine crackers
- 1/2 cup ice cream
- 1/3 to 1/2 cup frozen yogurt

1 serving of Meat:
- 1/4 cup cottage cheese
- 1/4 cup tuna or salmon
- 1 oz. cheese
- 1 scrambled egg
- 1 oz. chopped meat
- 4 oz. tofu

1 serving of Milk:
- 1/2 cup eggnog (no alcohol)
- 1 cup milk
- 1/2 cup sugar-free instant breakfast drink
- 1 cup creamed soup
- 1/2 cup sugar-free pudding
- 1/2 cup baked custard
- 1 cup artificially sweetened yogurt

1 serving of Fruit:
- 1/2 cup juice
- 1 frozen fruit juice bar
- 1/2 cup regular soda
- 2 tsp. honey
- 1 cup Gatorade
- 1/2 cup canned peaches or pears
- 1/2 cup applesauce
- 1/4 cup regular gelatin

Photo at right:
Lunch 2

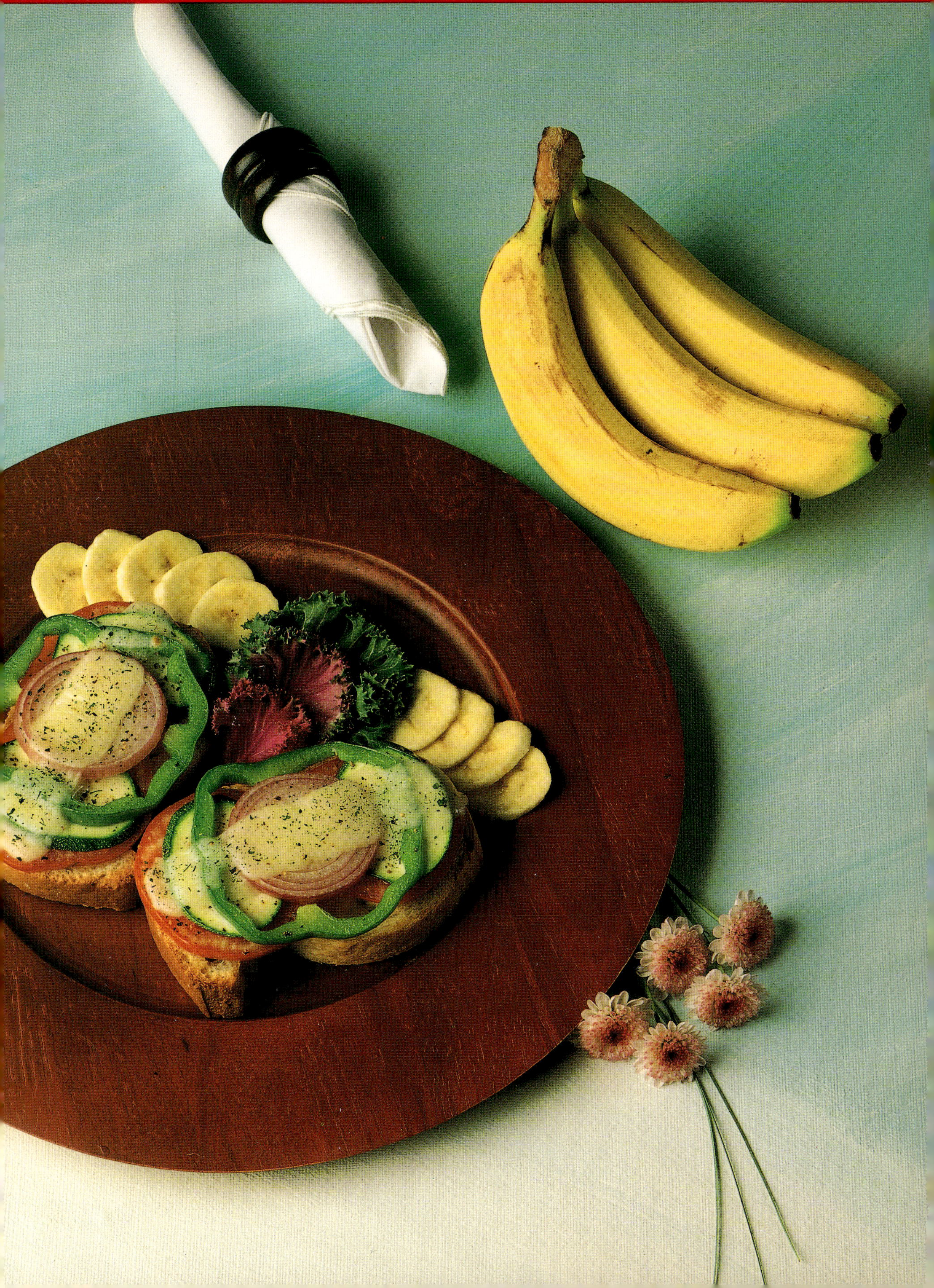

Each **breakfast** in this section has about **350 calories** and includes:

2	Starch/Bread	servings
1	Fruit	serving
1	Skim Milk	serving
1	Fat	serving

In some menus, one Meat serving has been used in place of either the Skim Milk serving or one of the Starch/Bread servings.

Each **lunch** in this section has about **450 calories** and includes:

2	Starch/Bread	servings
2	Meat	servings
0-1	Vegetable	serving
1	Fruit	serving
1	Fat	serving

In some menus, one Milk serving has been used in place of either one of the Meat or one of the Starch/Bread servings.

Each **dinner** in this section has about **550 calories** and includes:

2	Starch/Bread	servings
3	Meat	servings
1-2	Vegetable	servings
1	Fruit	serving
2	Fat	servings

In some menus, one Milk serving has been used in place of either one of the Meat or one of the Starch/Bread servings.

1

Tuna pocket:
- 1 7-inch pita, halved, stuffed with
- 1/2 cup shredded lettuce and
- 1/2 cup tuna salad made with
- 1 Tbsp. reduced-calorie mayonnaise

1/2 cup tomato juice
1/4 medium cantaloupe

BROILED OPEN-FACED VEGETARIAN SANDWICH
1 small banana

BROILED OPEN-FACED VEGETARIAN SANDWICH

Yield: 1 serving

Ingredients

2 slices Italian bread, cut 1-inch thick
1 Tbsp. reduced-calorie margarine
Zucchini slices
Tomato slices
Onion slices
Green pepper slices
Garlic powder
Basil
Pepper
2 oz. part-skim mozzarella cheese

Method

1. Spread Italian bread with 1 tsp. reduced-calorie margarine on each.
2. Top with tomato, zucchini, onion, and green pepper slices.
3. Sprinkle with garlic powder, basil, and pepper; top with cheese.
4. Broil until browned on edges and cheese is melted.

3

2 slices diet bread (40 calories each)
1 slice cold SPICY TURKEY LOAF
Lettuce or tomato slice or ketchup, if desired
1/2 mango or 12 cherries

SPICY TURKEY LOAF

Yield: 8 servings/Serving Size: 1 slice

Ingredients

1 1/2 lb. ground turkey
3/4 cup evaporated milk
1/4 cup finely chopped onion
1 cup bread crumbs
4 Tbsp. chili sauce
1/2 tsp. ground ginger
1/2 tsp. crushed fresh garlic clove
A few parsley or cilantro leaves, chopped

Method

1. Preheat oven to 350 degrees.
2. Mix all ingredients together. Press into an ungreased loaf pan.
3. Bake 45 minutes or until toothpick comes out clean. Cool about 5 minutes, then cut into 8 slices.

1 Arby's regular roast beef sandwich
Tossed salad with
2-3 Tbsp. fat-free salad dressing
1 orange

5

Stouffer's Lean Cuisine Cheese Cannelloni with Tomato Sauce
1/2 cup steamed broccoli with
1 tsp. regular margarine
2 bread sticks
1 cup mixed berries (strawberries, raspberries, blueberries)

LUNCH

6

Salad in a Pita:
1 1/2 cups tossed salad mixed with
1/4 cup low-fat cottage cheese and
1 Tbsp. reduced-calorie mayonnaise, placed into
1 7-inch whole-wheat pita and topped with
1/4 cup part-skim milk mozzarella cheese

4 raw apricots

7

1 package Lipton Cup-A-Soup Chicken Supreme*
4 RyKrisp crackers
Tossed salad with
1 oz. part-skim milk mozzarella cheese
1 oz. sliced turkey
2-3 Tbsp. fat-free salad dressing
2 plums

**High in sodium; for occasional use only.*

LUNCH

8

1 Burger King hamburger
Salad bar:
  1/2 cup mixed fruit
  1 cup raw vegetables, with greens
  1 Tbsp. salad dressing

1 1-1/2-oz. Provesta Meal-on-the-Go bar (available in sporting stores)
3 cups air-popped (fat-free) popcorn
2 tubes (2 oz. total) string cheese
1 cup carrot sticks
2 dried apple rings

1/2 ham sandwich:
- 1 slice bread with
- 1 oz. sliced ham,
- Lettuce and tomato, and
- 1 tsp. mayonnaise

2 pear halves, canned in juice and drained
1/4 cup nonfat or low-fat cottage cheese
4 RyKrisp crackers

11

Mexican chicken burrito:

- 1 10-inch soft tortilla
- 2 oz. leftover chicken, diced (1 thigh)
- 1 Tbsp. chopped fresh or dried dill
- Chopped onion and tomato, as desired
- 1 Tbsp. ranch salad dressing

2 tangerines

LUNCH

12

2 PIZZA MUFFINS

Tossed salad with
2 Tbsp. reduced-calorie salad dressing
1 apple

Yield: 12 muffins/Serving Size: 2 muffins

Ingredients

1 egg
1/2 cup tomato sauce
1 cup buttermilk or plain low-fat yogurt
1 tsp. dried oregano
1/4 tsp. garlic powder
1/4 tsp. freshly ground pepper
4 oz. mozzarella cheese, diced
1 1/2 cups whole-wheat flour
3 Tbsp. wheat germ
2 tsp. baking powder
1 tsp. baking soda
Sliced tomatoes and sesame seeds for garnish
Nonstick vegetable cooking spray

(Continued on page 49)

13

2 cups torn lettuce with:
- 1/2 cup tuna (canned in water)
- 1 chopped tomato
- 1/2 cup new potatoes, boiled, chopped, and chilled
- 5 small black, green, or Greek olives
- 2-3 Tbsp. fat-free salad dressing

6 saltine crackers
1 small pear

LUNCH

14

1 serving TORTILLA SOUP
Tossed salad with
2 Tbsp. reduced-calorie salad dressing
3 medium prunes

TORTILLA SOUP

Yield: 2 servings/Serving Size: 1 cup

Ingredients
3 6-inch flour tortillas, cut in
  1/2-inch strips
1 4-oz. can whole tomatoes
1/2 small onion, chopped
1/2 clove garlic, chopped
2 cups chicken broth
1/4 tsp. salt
1 Tbsp. cilantro
2 Tbsp. Monterey Jack cheese, shredded
Nonstick vegetable cooking spray

(Continued on page 49)

15

5 oz. sugar-free nonfat frozen yogurt
1/3 cup roasted sunflower seeds
1/2 cup Kellogg's All-Bran with extra fiber
1/2 banana

LUNCH

16

1 piece Kentucky Fried Chicken skinless center breast
1 ear corn-on-the-cob
1 medium apple
1 serving coleslaw

This menu is 1 fat exchange over the lunch allowance and is for occasional use only. Try to balance this meal with less fat at another meal that day.

17

1 serving FIESTA RICE
1/2 cup green beans
3 medium prunes
Tossed salad
1 Tbsp. creamy ranch dressing

FIESTA RICE

Yield: 4 servings/Serving Size: 1 cup

Ingredients

2 1/2 cups brown rice, cooked
3/4 cup low-fat (1%) cottage cheese
1 cup low-fat cheddar cheese, grated
2-oz. jar pimientos, drained and chopped
1/2 cup skim milk
1 large tomato, peeled and diced
Dash paprika
Nonstick vegetable cooking spray

Method

1. Preheat oven to 350 degrees.
2. Combine 1/2 cup of cheddar cheese and all other ingredients except paprika. Stir until well mixed.
3. Spray casserole with nonstick vegetable cooking spray.
4. Pour in mixture; top with remaining cheddar cheese and sprinkle well with paprika.
5. Bake 25 to 30 minutes.

LUNCH

18

Banana hot dog sandwich:
1 hot dog bun with
1/2 banana and
2 Tbsp. peanut butter

19

2 halves FAJITA IN A PITA
2 small tangerines

FAJITA IN A PITA

Yield: 4 servings

Ingredients

1/3 cup oil-free Italian salad dressing
1/3 cup low-sodium soy sauce
4 4-oz. chicken breast halves, skinned and boned
1 medium red pepper
1 medium yellow pepper
1 medium onion, sliced into rings
4 7-inch pitas, halved
1/4 cup plain low-fat yogurt
1/2 cup salsa
Nonstick vegetable cooking spray

Method

1. Combine salad dressing, soy sauce, and chicken in a 1-qt. casserole dish. Cover and chill at least 8 hours.

(Continued on page 51)

20

Stouffer's Beef Teriyaki with Rice and Vegetables
1 orange

21

1 serving SQUASH CASSEROLE
1/2 cup mixed citrus fruit sections

SQUASH CASSEROLE

Yield: 6 servings/Serving Size: 1/6 recipe

Ingredients

1 1/2 lb. yellow squash, sliced
2 Tbsp. margarine
1 cup shredded carrots
3 cups Pepperidge Farm stuffing mix
1 medium onion, chopped
1 cup reduced-calorie sour cream
1 egg
1 cup chicken broth or enough to moisten
12 oz. skinless turkey breast, cubed
Nonstick vegetable cooking spray

Method

1. Preheat oven to 375 degrees.
2. Saute onion in margarine.
3. Mix all ingredients.
4. Pour into a 2-qt. baking dish that has been sprayed with nonstick vegetable cooking spray.
5. Bake 30 to 40 minutes or until bubbly.

22

1-oz. package dry-roasted peanuts
2 tubes string cheese
6 to 8 Ryvita crackers
4 oz. tomato juice
1 medium apple or pear

1 TOMATO-CHEESE BAKE SANDWICH
15 grapes

TOMATO-CHEESE BAKE SANDWICH

Yield: 1 serving

Ingredients

2 slices whole-wheat bread
2 slices American cheese
4 slices tomato
6 green pepper strips
1 Tbsp. reduced-calorie salad dressing
Dash of oregano

Method

1. Top each slice of bread with 2 slices of tomato, 3 strips of green pepper, and half of the salad dressing. Place 1 slice of cheese over the dressing and sprinkle with oregano.
2. Broil until cheese is melted.

24

Lean Cuisine Glazed Chicken with Vegetable Rice
1/2 cup MARINATED CUCUMBERS
5 oz. sugar-free low-fat frozen yogurt

MARINATED CUCUMBERS

Yield: 4 servings/Serving Size: 1/2 cup

Ingredients

1/4 cup vinegar
2 Tbsp. water
1/4 tsp. salt
Dash paprika
Dash pepper
1 medium cucumber, peeled and sliced
1 medium onion, sliced and separated into rings
1 tsp. fresh parsley, minced

Method

1. Combine all ingredients.
2. Chill, stirring occasionally.

25

2 oz. cheddar cheese
4 bread sticks
1 medium apple

LUNCH

26

1 Taco Bell beef burrito or enchirito
1 apple

27

Stuffed baked potato:
- 1 medium baked potato topped with
- 2 oz. American cheese and
- 1/4 cup chopped broccoli

1 nectarine

LUNCH

28

McDonald's chicken salad with
2 Tbsp. Oriental salad dressing
1 small order of French fries

Breakfast #2 (Continued)
DOUBLE CORN MUFFINS
Method
1. Preheat oven to 375 degrees. Spray muffin tin with nonstick vegetable cooking spray or line with baking cups.
2. In a large bowl, stir together flour, cornmeal, sugar, baking powder, and salt.
3. In a small bowl, beat eggs and cottage or ricotta cheese until smooth; stir in corn.
4. Add wet mixture to dry ingredients; stir until just blended. Fill muffin cups two-thirds full.
5. Bake for 25 to 30 minutes. Serve warm.

Breakfast #6 (Continued)
TOFU GARDEN QUICHE
Method
1. Preheat oven to 325 degrees. Melt the margarine in a large skillet. Add onion and cook until onion is soft, about 5 minutes.
2. Add cooked vegetables and mix. Remove from heat and set aside.
3. Put eggs and half of the tofu into a blender and blend until smooth and creamy. Add remaining ingredients except vegetable mixture and cheese and blend until smooth.
4. Pour the tofu mixture into a large quiche dish or pie pan.
5. Sprinkle with Parmesan cheese.
6. Bake for 50 minutes to 1 hour or until knife comes out clean.

Lunch #12 (Continued)
PIZZA MUFFINS
Method
1. Preheat oven to 400 degrees. Spray muffin tin with nonstick vegetable cooking spray or line with baking cups.
2. Blend the egg, tomato sauce, and buttermilk or yogurt with a mixer or food processor. Add the spices. Add the cheese, reserving 1/4 cup for topping.
3. In another bowl, mix the flour, wheat germ, baking powder, and baking soda.
4. Combine the two mixtures until flour is no longer visible. Spoon batter into muffin tin, filling each well about 2/3 full. Top each muffin with a slice of tomato and some cheese; sprinkle with sesame seeds.
5. Bake 20 to 25 minutes.

Lunch #14 (Continued)
TORTILLA SOUP
Method
1. Fry tortilla strips in heated skillet well coated with nonstick vegetable cooking spray.
2. Puree tomatoes, onions, and garlic.
3. Bring chicken broth to a boil in a 2-qt. saucepan. Stir in tomato puree, salt, and cilantro. Reduce heat and simmer for 10 minutes.
4. Add half of the tortilla strips to soup.
5. Garnish with cheese and remaining tortilla strips to serve.

Dinner #1 (Continued)
HURRY-UP BEEF STEW
Method
1. Spray pressure cooker with nonstick vegetable cooking spray.
2. Brown the meat over medium-high heat. Remove fat.
3. Remove the meat; put the pressure-cooker trivet in the bottom of the cooker. Return the meat to the cooker.
4. Add all remaining ingredients.
5. Cover, bring to pressure, and simmer at pressure for 30 minutes.
6. Turn off heat and let pressure reduce by itself.
7. When pressure has returned to normal, open carefully and remove bay leaf.
8. Stir contents.

Dinner #3 (Continued)
SMOTHERED CHICKEN
Method
1. In a deep saucepan or Dutch oven, brown chicken parts in oil, then pour off excess oil.
2. Add onion, garlic, and spices.
3. Cover chicken with water. Cover pot and bring to a boil, then lower heat and simmer for about 2 1/2 to 3 hours.
4. Add carrots and peas. Cover pot; bring back to a boil, then lower heat and simmer for another 20 to 30 minutes.

Breakfast #9 (Continued)
PEANUT BUTTER AND JELLY MUFFINS
Method
1. Preheat oven to 350 degrees.
2. Spray muffin tin with nonstick vegetable cooking spray or line with baking cups.
3. In a large bowl, mix flour, sugar and baking powder.
4. In another bowl, beat peanut butter and egg until smooth. Add milk a little at a time, stirring after each addition.
5. Pour peanut butter mixture over dry ingredients; fold in with a rubber spatula just until dry ingredients are moistened. Batter will be stiff.
6. Spoon 2 scant Tbsp. batter into each muffin cup and smooth the surface out to the top edge of the cup. Then top each muffin with a heaping tsp. of fruit spread; cover with 2 more Tbsp. of batter.
7. Bake 20 to 25 minutes or until lightly browned.

Breakfast #10 (Continued)
IOWA CORN PANCAKES
Method
1. Combine milk, oats, and corn in a large mixing bowl and let stand for 8 minutes.
2. Mix flours, salt, and baking soda in a small bowl and set aside.
3. Add egg substitute to milk mixture and beat until blended.
4. Add dry ingredients to wet ingredients and stir until just mixed.
5. Pour slightly less than 1/3 cup batter on a hot griddle that has been sprayed with nonstick vegetable cooking spray.
6. Cook until bubbles form on edges and edges start to dry.
7. Turn and cook 2 to 3 more minutes.

Breakfast #16 (Continued)
QUICK HOMEMADE RAISIN BREAD
Method
1. Preheat oven to 350 degrees. Spray a 9 by 5-inch loaf pan with nonstick vegetable cooking spray and lightly dust with flour.
2. Combine raisins and water; set aside for 30 minutes.
3. In a large bowl, combine flour, baking soda, artificial sweetener, cinnamon, and salt. Add raisins with liquid, egg, vanilla, and oil.
4. Mix just until dry ingredients are moistened.
5. Pour into loaf pan. Bake for 40 to 45 minutes or until golden brown and firm to the touch.
6. Let stand 5 minutes. Serve warm.

Breakfast #19 (Continued)
SUGARLESS BLUEBERRY MUFFINS
Method
1. Preheat oven to 400 degrees. Spray muffin tin with nonstick vegetable cooking spray or line with baking cups.
2. Lightly coat the blueberries with 2 tsp. flour by shaking together in a paper bag.
3. In a large bowl, stir together 1 3/4 cups flour, baking powder, nutmeg, and cinnamon.
4. In a small bowl, beat the eggs lightly. Add oil, orange juice, and grated rind.
5. Add the liquid to the dry mixture and stir gently. Before the two mixtures are fully combined, fold in the blueberries.
6. Fill each muffin cup about 2/3 full. Bake 20 to 25 minutes.

Breakfast #20 (Continued)
SWEET POTATO-RAISIN COOKIES
Method
1. Preheat oven to 350 degrees. Soak raisins in hot water to cover for 5 minutes, then drain.
2. Cream margarine, then add sweet potatoes, egg, and vanilla; beat until creamy.
3. Mix flour, allspice, salt, nutmeg, baking soda, baking powder, and cinnamon. Add to creamed mixture and mix well.
4. Add raisins, nuts, and bran.
5. Drop onto cookie sheet that has been sprayed with nonstick vegetable cooking spray.
6. Bake for 12 minutes or until done.

Breakfast #24 (Continued)
VEGETABLE FRITTATA
Method
1. Preheat oven to 350 degrees.
2. Whisk eggs with egg whites and set aside.
3. Spray medium saucepan with nonstick vegetable cooking spray. Add oil.
4. Over medium-high heat, saute vegetables for 5 to 7 minutes.
5. Place sauteed vegetables into a baking dish sprayed with nonstick vegetable cooking spray. Pour blended eggs onto sauteed vegetables and sprinkle cheese on top.
6. Bake frittata for 12 to 15 minutes (or keep in saute pan and cook on stove top over low heat for 10 to 12 minutes).

Breakfast #26 (Continued)
SPICY ZUCCHINI BARS
Method
1. Preheat oven to 350 degrees.
2. Combine flour, baking powder, baking soda, cinnamon, cloves, and salt in a medium bowl.
3. In a large bowl, combine eggs, oil, sugar, yogurt, and vanilla; beat well.
4. Stir in zucchini and raisins; add flour mixture and stir until moistened.
5. Pour into a 13 by 9 by 2-inch baking dish coated with nonstick vegetable cooking spray.
6. Bake for 30 minutes or until toothpick comes out clean. Cool in pan.
7. Sprinkle with powdered sugar and bran flakes and cut into bars.

Breakfast #28 (Continued)
BAKED RICE PUDDING
Method
1. Preheat oven to 325 degrees.
2. Heat milk in the top of a double boiler over simmering water until surface begins to wrinkle.
3. Blend together the eggs, sugar, salt, and vanilla. Add hot milk gradually, stirring to mix well.
4. Add rice. Pour into four 6-oz. individual custard cups. Sprinkle surface lightly with nutmeg.
5. Set cups in a deep pan; pour hot water around cups to come to within 1/2 inch of tops of cups.
6. Bake 50 to 60 minutes or until toothpick comes out clean.
7. Remove from heat and water pan. Chill for several hours before serving.
8. Sprinkle with artificial sweetener, if desired.

Lunch #19 (Continued)
FAJITA IN A PITA
2. Remove chicken from marinade, reserving marinade.
3. Grill chicken, covered, over medium hot coals for 5 minutes on each side. Cut chicken into strips and keep warm.
4. Coat a nonstick skillet with nonstick vegetable cooking spray. Place over medium-high heat. Saute pepper and onion for 3 minutes.
5. Add 3 Tbsp. marinade. Cook until vegetables are tender but crisp and liquid is absorbed.
6. Fill pita halves with chicken strips and vegetables. Serve with yogurt and salsa.

Dinner #4 (Continued)
LIGHT AND CREAMY YOGURT PIE
Yield: 8 servings/Serving Size: 1/8 recipe

Ingredients
- 1 package low-fat whipped topping (equal to 8 oz. or 1 cup)
- 1 cup nonfat yogurt with artificial sweetener
- 2 cups sliced strawberries or 1 1/2 cups other fruit
- 1 store-bought graham cracker crust

Method
1. Make whipped topping according to package directions.
2. Fold in yogurt and most of the fruit. Fill crust.
3. Garnish with remaining fruit. Chill or freeze.
4. May be served frozen.

Dinner #8 (Continued)
NEW ENGLAND CHICKEN CROQUETTES
Method
1. Preheat oven to 375 degrees.
2. Melt margarine over low heat; stir in flour until smooth. Add milk gradually, whisk until smooth; add Worcestershire sauce, chervil, salt, pepper, and chicken. Cool.
3. When cold, form into 8 balls using 1/3 cup mixture per ball.
4. Roll in bread crumbs, egg, and again in bread crumbs.
5. Place on cookie sheet well sprayed with nonstick vegetable cooking spray. Bake for 25 to 30 minutes until light golden brown.

Dinner #12 (Continued)

MEATLESS CHILI

Method

1. Combine all ingredients in an 8-qt. stockpot. Bring to a boil.
2. Reduce to medium heat and cook partially covered for 3 to 3 1/2 hours, stirring occasionally.

Dinner #13 (Continued)

SEASONED GREENS

Yield: 8 servings/Serving Size: 1/2 cup

Ingredients

1 large bunch of collard, mustard, or turnip greens or 1 lb. of frozen greens
2 fresh center-cut pork chops, fat trimmed, chopped
Salt, pepper, and hot sauce to taste (optional)

Method

1. Rinse greens well in water. Cut or tear into small pieces. Peel and cut turnips, if included.
2. Place greens and chopped pork in a 2-qt. pan and cover with water. Bring to a boil and cook about 5 minutes.

Dinner #19 (Continued)

BROCCOLI CORN CHOWDER

Method

1. In a large kettle, combine chicken broth, broccoli, and corn.
2. Bring to a boil. Reduce heat to low and simmer 15 minutes. Set aside.
3. Saute the mushrooms and onion in the margarine.
4. Blend the flour and pepper into the mushroom mixture. Add to broccoli mixture.
5. Add milk and simmer over low heat for about 30 minutes, stirring occasionally.
6. Stir in pimientos before serving.

Dinner #20 (Continued)

SAUCY SEAFOOD STIR FRY

Method

1. Spray a large frying pan or wok with nonstick vegetable cooking spray; heat to medium high.
2. Stir fry broccoli, cauliflower, and carrots about 4 minutes. Sprinkle with water if they start to burn. Then add peppers.
3. Add shrimp to mixture and continue heating until shrimp turn pink. Add scallops and continue heating until scallops turn white. Set aside.
4. Melt margarine in microwave or oven. Whip mayonnaise and melted margarine together until smooth. Add lemon juice.
5. Combine with stir fry mixture.

WALDORF SALAD

Yield: 6 servings/Serving Size: 1/2 cup

Ingredients

2 large apples, cored and diced
2 tsp. lemon juice
1 cup diced celery
6 Tbsp. walnuts, coarsely chopped
1/4 cup dark or golden raisins
3 Tbsp. mayonnaise
2 Tbsp. skim milk
Lettuce leaves

Method

1. Put the apples in a medium bowl and add lemon juice. Toss.
2. Mix the celery, walnuts, and raisins in a small bowl.
3. Beat the mayonnaise and milk together until smooth. Add the the celery mixture.
4. Toss with the apple mixture.
5. Serve chilled on lettuce leaves.

Dinner #21 (Continued)
CLAM SAUCE
Method

1. Heat skillet and add olive oil.
2. Saute onion, pepper, and mushrooms. Add clams and liquid.
3. Simmer to reduce liquid by 1/3 to 1/2.
4. Add tomato and cream and simmer until large glossy bubbles form.
5. Season and toss with grated cheese.
6. Serve 1/5 of recipe over 1 cup of cooked linguine.

Dinner #25 (Continued)
CHICKEN CURRY
Method

1. Make a paste of the gingerroot, garlic, and 2 Tbsp. of water.
2. Saute onion in corn oil until brown. Add all the spices and the chicken and yogurt; continue to cook, sprinkling with additional water as required to keep from sticking.
3. Cook until chicken browns (about 10 minutes). Add 1 cup of water and let simmer on low heat for about 45 minutes or until chicken is tender.
4. Add chopped tomato after about 30 minutes. Before serving, add chopped cilantro leaves.

Photo at right:
60-Calorie Snacks 6, 15, and 18

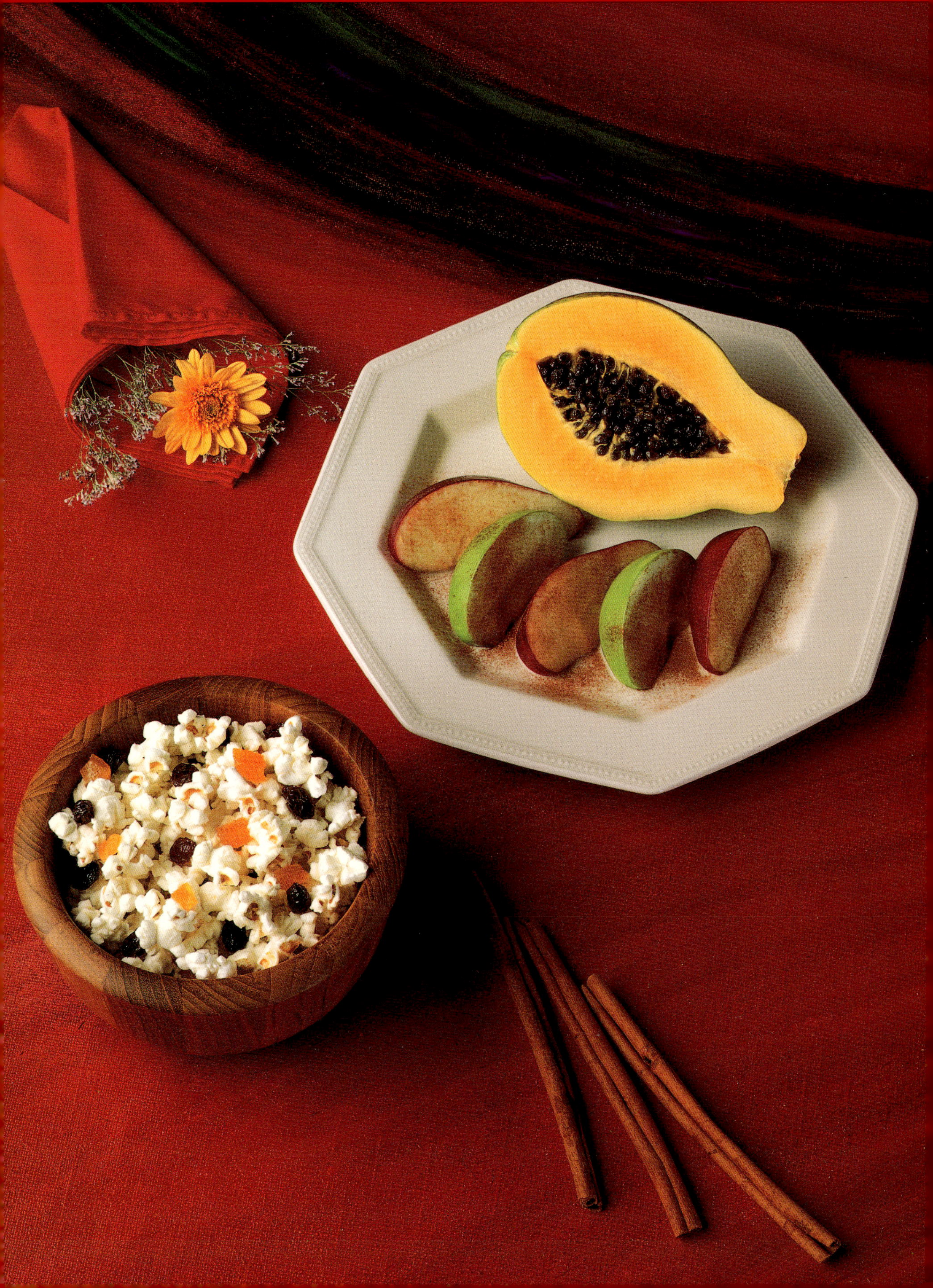

The snacks in this section are divided into three groups:

Each **60-calorie** snack equals	1 Fruit **OR** 1 Starch/Bread serving
Each **125-calorie** snack equals	1 Starch/Bread serving **AND** 1 Fat serving
Each **170-calorie** snack equals	1 Starch/Bread serving **AND** 1 Skim Milk **OR** 1 Meat serving

60 calories

1
1/2 cup fruit juice

2
3 pretzel rods

3
1 fat-free mini muffin

4
15 FROSTY GRAPES

FROSTY GRAPES
Yield: 4 servings
Serving Size: 15 grapes

Ingredients
1 lb. seedless grapes
1 3-oz. package of lime sugar-free gelatin powder

Method
1. Divide grapes into small bunches. Rinse and drain.
2. Put gelatin powder in a container with a lid that can be frozen. Add grapes and shake to coat. Shake off excess powder from grape bunches.
3. Put lid on container and freeze. Serve frozen.

5
Mixed dried fruit: 1 apple ring, 1 apricot half, 1 prune

6
1/2 papaya with fresh lime juice

7
2/3 cup fruit-flavored, sugar-free, nonfat yogurt

8
7 mini rice and popcorn cakes

9
3 RyKrisp crackers

10
2 Chinese fortune cookies

11
1/2 cup fruit juice mixed with 1/2 cup sparkling water

12
1 package (0.75 oz.) Sunkist Fruit Roll

13
4 oz. unsweetened applesauce

14
1/2 frozen banana on a stick dipped in 2 Tbsp. CHOCOLATE-FLAVORED SYRUP

CHOCOLATE-FLAVORED SYRUP
Yield: 15 servings
Serving Size: 2 Tbsp.

Ingredients
1/2 cup dry cocoa, firmly packed
1 1/2 cups cold water
1/4 tsp. salt
Artificial sweetener to substitute for 1/2 cup sugar
2 1/2 tsp. vanilla

Method
1. Mix cocoa, water, and salt in a heavy saucepan until smooth. Bring to a boil and simmer gently, stirring constantly, for 3 minutes.
2. Remove from heat and let cool 10 minutes.
3. Add artificial sweetener and vanilla and mix well.
4. Store refrigerated in a jar. Stir well in jar before measuring to use.

15
cinnamon apple wedges
(Cut 1 small apple into wedges and sprinkle with a mixture of cinnamon and artificial sweetener.)

16
watermelon pops
(Cut 1 1/4 cups of watermelon into big chunks and insert wooden sticks in each chunk. Wrap in plastic wrap and freeze. Eat frozen.)

17
1 yogurt pop
(Punch a wooden stick through the lid of a 5-oz. cup of sugar-free fruit-flavored yogurt. Freeze.)

18
1 cup air-popped popcorn mixed with
1 Tbsp. chopped dried mixed fruit or raisins

19
5 pudding kisses
(Drop by level tablespoons 1/3 cup of artificially sweetened chocolate pudding onto wax paper. Freeze. Makes 5 kisses.)

20
2 pear halves, canned in juice and drained

21
1 fresh navel orange

125 calories

1
1 mini-bagel with 1 Tbsp. regular cream cheese

2
2 Salerno dinosaur graham crackers

3
6 cups microwaved Orville Redenbacher's Lite popcorn

4
1 Nature Valley granola bar (2 bars per package)

5
4 RyKrisp crackers, divided into 12 sections, with cheese spread (*Combine 1 1/2 Tbsp. of reduced-calorie cream cheese with 1 tsp. dried onion flakes.*) topped with cucumber, red pepper, and green onion slices

6
1/2 cup blanched sugar snap peas (*Dip washed and stringed pea pods in boiling water for 1 minute; drain promptly and plunge into ice water to chill.*) with
2 Tbsp. reduced-calorie ranch dressing for dipping

7
Celery sticks spread with
1 1/2 Tbsp. no-sugar-added peanut butter

8
1/2 cup sugar-free low-fat frozen yogurt

9
27 Sunshine Cheez-It crackers

10
1/3 cup Pepperidge Farm Goldfish crackers

11
1 SWEET POTATO-RAISIN COOKIE
(see Breakfast 20)
3/4 cup skim milk

12
1/2 medium potato with
1 Tbsp. light margarine

13
1/2 medium baked acorn or butternut squash with
1 tsp. margarine and cinnamon and artificial sweetener to taste

14
1/3 cup BLACK BEAN DIP with vegetable chips (sliced raw carrots, cauliflower, broccoli, and celery)

BLACK BEAN DIP

Yield: 2 cups
Serving Size: 1/3 cup

Ingredients

1 15-oz. can black beans, drained
1 small onion, chopped
1 small green pepper
1 clove garlic, chopped
1 1/2 Tbsp. red wine vinegar
1 1/2 Tbsp. olive oil
1/2 tsp. sugar
Salt, pepper, hot sauce to taste

Method

1. Combine all ingredients in a food processor.
2. Process, pushing off and on until beans are coarsely mashed.
3. Season to taste.

15
1 Kellogg's Eggo apple cinnamon waffle with
2 Tbsp. Cary's sugar-free syrup

16
1 pita garlic toast (*Split pita into 2 flat rounds; spread 1 round with 1 Tbsp. reduced-calorie margarine and sprinkle lightly with garlic powder and Parmesan cheese, then toast.*)

17
6 Nabisco Triscuits, dipped in
1/4 cup salsa

18
6 small vanilla wafers
1/2 cup diet cherry gelatin
1 Tbsp. whipped topping

19
3 Wasa crackers spread with
2 Tbsp. reduced-calorie cream cheese mixed with
2 tsp. salsa

20
14 chocolate Nabisco Teddy Grahams

21
1/2 cup Nabisco doo dads snack mix

170 calories

1
1 1-oz. bag Nabisco Teddy Grahams
8 oz. sugar-free hot cocoa

2
2 Nabisco Lorna Doone shortbread cookies and
1 cup skim or 1% milk

3
3 oz. fresh crab and
1 tsp. reduced-calorie mayonnaise spread on
3 slices cocktail-size pumpernickel bread

4
3/4 cup General Mills Triples cereal
1 cup skim or 1% milk

5
1/2 bagel with
1 Tbsp. peanut butter

6
1 1.5-oz. Provesta Meal-on-the-Go bar (available in sporting stores)

7
Skins of 2 baked potatoes *(Split baked potatoes in half and scoop out all but 1/8 to 1/4 inch of potato flesh; sprinkle with 1 oz. grated part-skim mozzarella cheese and paprika, then bake in 450-degree oven or broil until cheese melts and bubbles.)*

8
2 thin slices pumpernickel bread (1 oz. total)
1 oz. thinly sliced ham
2 tsp. reduced-calorie cream cheese *(Spread ham with cream cheese and roll up, then slice thinly and arrange on bread.)*

9
1 oz. pickled herring on
3 slices cocktail-size rye bread

10
1 oz. string cheese
4 Nabisco Triscuits

11
1 serving BAKED RICE PUDDING
(see Breakfast 28)

12
2/3 cup HOPPIN' JOHN
(see Dinner 13)

13
2 by 2 by 1-inch piece of cornbread
1/2 cup skim or 1% milk

14
11.5-oz. can of tomato juice
3/4 oz. sunflower seeds

15
1/4 cup low-fat cottage cheese mixed with
1 tsp. dry diet fruit-flavored gelatin powder
6 saltine crackers

16
2 rice and popcorn cakes
1 oz. cheese spread (Cheez Whiz or Alouette)

17
1/2 English muffin
1 oz. low-fat Alpine Lace for mozzarella lovers

18
8 oz. sugar-free fruit-flavored yogurt
3 graham cracker squares

19
1 slice Little Caesar's cheese pizza
diet soda

20
1/4 cup low-fat cottage cheese with
1 Tbsp. chives
6 herb-flavored crackers

21
1/2 cup sugar-free banana pudding with
3 crushed thin chocolate wafers

Photo at right:
Barbecue Lunch 2

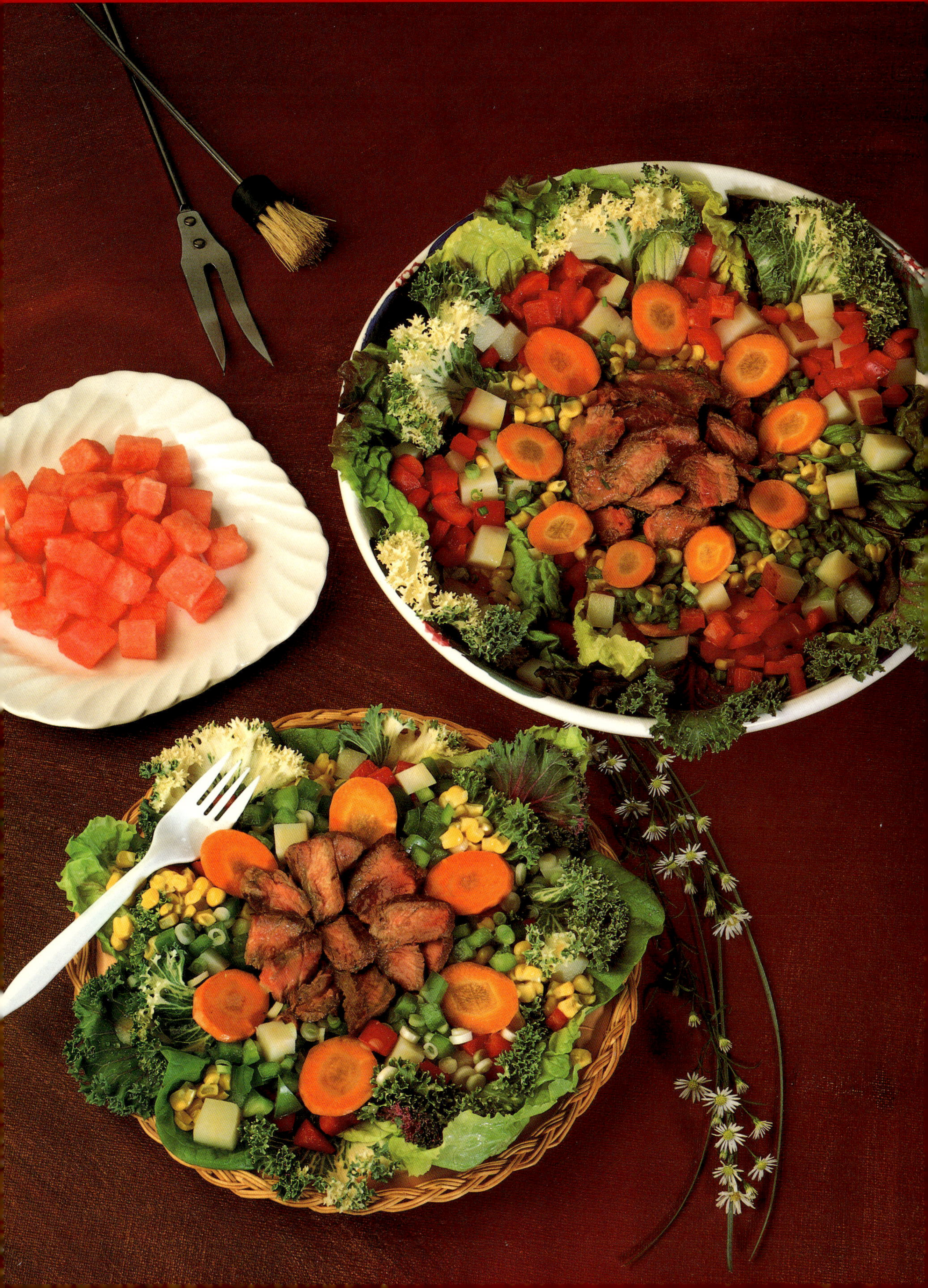

PICNICS & BARBECUES

Whatever the weather, picnics and barbecues are in season. In some families, it wouldn't be summer without the family chef working over a grill of hot coals. In other families, fall or spring means a canoe trip and a picnic lunch at an inviting spot along the way. Perhaps your traditions include birthdays celebrated with a picnic in the zoo or yearly beach barbecues with friends. You get to enjoy the company of family and friends for a meal, plus you have a chance to stretch your legs on a hike and go for a swim. Don't let rain dampen your spirits—just lay out your picnic in front of the fireplace and set up some board games.

Will it be hard to maintain your meal plan? No! With a little advance planning, you'll be able to avoid the temptation of the typical high-fat, high-calorie picnic foods. The extra planning and effort it takes to create these special occasions is well worth the added fun of eating special picnic and barbecue foods outdoors.

In the following pages, we offer helpful tips and tasty menus for meals that you can prepare for backyard barbecuing or for easy satisfying picnics. Some even include convenience foods you can pick up on the way to your picnic.

And by the way, even if it's cold and snowy outside, these meals taste just as good indoors.

Tips for Good Nutrition

- Use fish, poultry, or lean red meat. Fish that tends to fall apart can be contained in foil or special wire baskets.
- If eating beef or pork, use low-fat cuts such as tenderloin or round, sirloin, or flank steak and trim all excess fat.
- Make hamburgers from extralean ground beef, which contains less than 15 percent fat. There are even ground beef products with less than 10 percent fat. Adding shredded vegetables to your hamburger mixture will increase the nutrition and decrease calories.
- Use reduced-calorie or no-oil salad dressings and "light" mayonnaise or nonfat plain yogurt in salads.

Tips for Good Health

- Never put cooked food back onto a plate that held raw meat. Raw meat contains bacteria that are destroyed while cooking—placing cooked meat on a plate that held raw meat could recontaminate it.
- Contrary to popular belief, adding mayonnaise to salads helps preserve them by slowing bacterial growth; however, they still need to be kept cold.
- Foods with cream filling or salads with eggs spoil easily and can cause food poisoning.
- Keep food in a cooler in the shade.

Tips for Good Eating

- Marinate vegetables and meats overnight before grilling to enhance flavor and tenderness. An easy marinade (or salad dressing) is 2 parts vinegar (try a flavored one) to 1 part oil with your favorite herbs.

- Wait to place food on the grill until the flames have died and the coals are white.

- Use the leftover marinade for basting while you cook, but note that if it has been exposed to raw meat, it should be cooked before eating.

- Do not puncture the meat when turning it—this lets juices escape. Use tongs instead.

PICNIC LUNCHES

1

1/2 cup deli pasta salad made with raw vegetables and Italian dressing
6 Nabisco Triscuits
2 oz. skim mozzarella cheese
4 dried apple rings

2

2 1-oz. slices of French bread
2 oz. Monterey Jack (or other favorite) cheese
1/4 bell pepper, cut in strips
1/4 cucumber, cut in spears
15 grapes
Sparkling mineral water

3

2 barbecued chicken wings (from deli)
1/2 cup CORN RELISH
1/4 cup baked beans
Assorted raw vegetables dipped in
1 Tbsp. ranch dressing mixed with
1 Tbsp. nonfat plain yogurt
1 1 by 5-inch slice watermelon

CORN RELISH

Yield: 6 servings
Serving Size: 1/2 cup

Ingredients
2 cups whole-kernel corn
1/2 green pepper, chopped
1/2 red pepper, chopped
1/2 cup red onion, chopped
1 1/2 Tbsp. oil
1/4 cup vinegar
3 or 4 packets artificial sweetener
Dash cumin

Method
1. Mix together all ingredients.
2. Chill 2 hours.

PICNIC DINNERS

1 piece cold OVEN-FRIED CHICKEN
2/3 cup HEALTHY POTATO SALAD
1/2 cup ROGER'S COLESLAW
2-3 tomato slices
1 1/4 cup fresh strawberries, whole
FRESH LEMONADE

OVEN-FRIED CHICKEN

Yield: 4 servings
Serving size: 1 piece

Ingredients

4 small chicken breasts (or 4 medium legs or thighs)
2/3 cup whole-wheat flour
1/2 tsp. paprika
1/2 tsp. salt
1/2 tsp. pepper
4 Tbsp. low-fat milk
4 tsp. melted margarine or oil

Method

1. Remove skin from chicken.
2. Combine flour with other dry ingredients.
3. Mix margarine or oil and milk.
4. Dip chicken in milk mixture, then dredge in flour mixture.
5. Place chicken in nonstick baking dish.
6. Bake at 350 degrees for 20 to 30 minutes or until golden brown.

HEALTHY POTATO SALAD

Yield: 4 servings
Serving size: 2/3 cup

Ingredients

2 medium potatoes
1 egg, hardboiled
1/4 cup celery, chopped
1/4 cup green pepper, chopped
1/4 cup sweet onion or scallions, chopped
2 Tbsp. pimiento, chopped
1 Tbsp. prepared mustard
3 Tbsp. Kraft Free nonfat mayonnaise dressing

Method

1. Cut potatoes into small half-inch cubes, leaving skin on. Boil in lightly salted water until cooked (8 to 10 minutes). Drain.
2. Combine all ingredients.
3. Refrigerate until served.

PICNIC DINNERS

ROGER'S COLESLAW

Yield: 8 servings
Serving size: 1/2 cup

Ingredients

1 lb. head of green cabbage, shredded
1 medium cucumber, peeled and chopped
1/2 cup reduced-calorie mayonnaise
1 Tbsp. vinegar
2 to 3 packets of Equal or other artificial sweetener
Dash salt
Pepper to taste
1 tsp. celery seed (optional)

Method

1. Combine all ingredients.
2. Refrigerate until served.

FRESH LEMONADE

Yield: 4 servings
Serving size: 1 cup

Ingredients

2/3 cup fresh lemon juice
3 1/3 cups water
Artificial sweetener to taste, but no more than equivalent to 1/2 cup sugar

Method

1. Mix all ingredients.
2. Chill and serve with ice.

PICNIC DINNERS

2

Hoagie:
- 1 2-oz. French roll
- 3 oz. total assorted cheeses or lunch meat
- Sliced tomatoes, lettuce, peppers, and onions
- Mustard to taste

1 serving FRESH TOMATO ASPIC
1 RASPBERRY FUDGE BROWNIE

FRESH TOMATO ASPIC

Yield: 6 servings
Serving Size: 1/6 recipe

Ingredients

2 cups fresh tomatoes, peeled, seeded, and finely chopped **(see Barbecue Dinner 3)**
1 envelope unflavored gelatin
2 tsp. balsamic or red wine vinegar
1/4 cup celery leaves, finely chopped
1/2 tsp. salt (optional)
1/4 tsp. pepper, fresly ground
6 lettuce leaves
2 Tbsp. reduced-calorie mayonnaise

Method

1. Place 1 cup of tomatoes in a small saucepan and sprinkle with gelatin. Bring to a boil over medium heat, stirring constantly, until gelatin is dissolved.
2. Remove from heat. Stir in remaining tomatoes, vinegar, celery leaves, salt, and pepper. Mix well and pour into a 7 by 3-inch nonstick loaf pan.
3. Cover and refrigerate until firm or overnight. Unmold. Slice and place on lettuce. Top each slice with a 1-tsp. dollop of reduced-calorie mayonnaise.

RASPBERRY FUDGE BROWNIES

Yield: 20 brownies
Serving Size: 1 brownie

Ingredients

1 10-oz. package of frozen raspberries in light syrup, thawed but not drained
1/4 cup plus 2 Tbsp. margarine
1/4 cup plus 2 Tbsp. unsweetened cocoa
1/2 cup sugar
2 eggs, beaten (or 1/2 cup egg substitute)
1/2 tsp. vanilla
1 1/2 cups flour
1/8 tsp. salt
Nonstick vegetable cooking spray

Method

1. Drain raspberries, reserving 3 Tbsp. juice. Set raspberries and juice aside.
2. Combine margarine and cocoa in a large saucepan. Cook over low heat, stirring constantly, until margarine melts and mixture becomes smooth. Remove from heat and let cool slightly.
3. Add sugar, eggs, and vanilla to cocoa mixture, stirring well. Combine flour and salt and add to cocoa mixture, folding in gently. Gently fold raspberries into cocoa mixture.
4. Spoon batter into an 8-inch square baking dish that has been coated with nonstick vegetable cooking spray. Bake at 350 degrees for 20 minutes or until toothpick comes out clean. Cut into 20 squares.

BARBECUE LUNCHES

1

1/2 cup Sloppy Joe filling on a
Reduced-calorie hamburger bun
1 serving GRILLED VEGGIES
1/2 cup MARINATED CUCUMBERS
(see Lunch 24)
1 serving STRAWBERRY SHORTCAKE

GRILLED VEGGIES

Yield: 1 serving

Ingredients
- 1/2 medium baking potato
- 1 carrot, sliced
- 1/2 medium onion, sliced
- 1 small summer squash, sliced
- Garlic salt
- Pepper
- 1 Tbsp. extralight margarine

Method
1. Place vegetables in an 8-inch square of heavy-duty aluminum foil.
2. Add seasonings and dot with margarine.
3. Grill about 30 minutes over low-heat coals.

STRAWBERRY SHORTCAKE

Yield: 8 servings
Serving size: 1/8 recipe

Ingredients
- 1/2 store-bought angelfood cake (7 oz.)
- 2 cups fresh strawberries, sliced
- 1 cup light whipped topping

Method
1. Cut cake into eight portions.
2. Place each slice of cake on a dessert dish and add 1/4 cup strawberries.
3. Top with 2 Tbsp. whipped topping.

BARBECUE LUNCHES

2

1 serving SUMMER MAIN-DISH SALAD
1 1/4 cups watermelon cubes

SUMMER MAIN-DISH SALAD

Yield: 4 servings
Serving Size: 1/4 recipe

Ingredients

1 cup frozen corn kernels
4 tsp. vegetable oil
3 garlic cloves, sliced
1/4 cup wine vinegar
1 Tbsp. Dijon mustard
/2 tsp. salt (optional)
1/8 tsp. pepper
1/4 tsp. sugar
12 oz. grilled sirloin, sliced
1 cup cooked potatoes, cubed
1 cup green onions, sliced
1/2 cup carrots, sliced thinly
1 cup red pepper, diced
1 cup green pepper, diced
Salad greens

Method

1. Cook corn according to package directions.
2. In a small saucepan, heat oil; saute garlic until golden brown.
3. Remove from heat and cool; strain and reserve oil; discard garlic.
4. In a large bowl, combine reserved oil, vinegar, mustard, salt, pepper, and sugar.
5. Combine oil mixture with corn, sirloin, potatoes, green onions, carrots, and both kinds of peppers. Mix well, cover, and chill.
6. Serve in a bowl lined with salad greens.

3

1 small French roll
2 oz. grilled turkey Italian sausage
1/4 cup marinara sauce
1 serving FRESH TOMATO AND BASIL SALAD
1 fresh peach

FRESH TOMATO AND BASIL SALAD

Yield: 4 servings
Serving Size: 4 tomato wedges

Ingredients

3/4 cup red wine vinegar
1 Tbsp. olive oil
1/4 tsp. garlic powder
1/8 tsp. pepper
1/4 tsp. salt (optional)
1/2 cup fresh basil, chopped
4 tomatoes

Method

1. Whisk together vinegar, oil, garlic powder, pepper, salt, and basil.
2. Cut each tomato into 4 wedges and pour dressing over them.
3. Marinate tomatoes for 3 to 4 hours.

BARBECUE DINNERS

1

1 serving GRILLED PICANTE CHICKEN
1/2 cup potato salad
Raw vegetables dipped in
Fat-free salad dressing
3/4 cup fresh pineapple, cubed

GRILLED PICANTE CHICKEN

Yield: 8 servings
Serving size: 1/2 breast

Ingredients

4 chicken breasts, skinned, boned, and cut in half
1 cup picante sauce
2 packets artificial sweetener
4 tsp. Dijon-style mustard

Method

1. Mix picante sauce, artificial sweetener, and mustard. Marinate chicken in this mixture for 4 to 8 hours in the refrigerator.
2. When coals are white, place chicken on the grill; turn after 5 minutes.
3. Brush on marinade while chicken cooks. Chicken should be done after a total of 15 to 20 minutes.

2

3 oz. beef Western rib, grilled and basted with
2 Tbsp. barbecue sauce
1 Pillsbury buttermilk or country style biscuit
1 cup steamed green beans flavored with
1 slice Canadian bacon, chopped
3 oz. Ore-Ida Zesties fries, baked
3/4 cup RASPBERRY-ORANGE GELATIN SUPREME

RASPBERRY-ORANGE GELATIN SUPREME

Yield: 6 servings
Serving Size: 3/4 cup

Ingredients

1 packet orange sugar-free gelatin
1 packet raspberry sugar-free gelatin
2 cups 100% raspberry juice
2 cups water
11 oz. mandarin orange sections, packed in light syrup

Method

1. Pour gelatin packets into a 2-qt. bowl.
2. In a small pan, mix raspberry juice with water and heat to boiling.
3. Mix boiling juice mixture into gelatin, stirring until gelatin is dissolved thoroughly.
4. Chill until thickened but not completely gelled. Add orange sections, stirring to spread throughout gelatin.
5. Chill until firm.

BARBECUE DINNERS

3

1 serving GAZPACHO
3 oz. swordfish grilled with
Green peppers and onions
2/3 cup MIXED-FIBER PILAF
1/2 papaya with
Lime juice

GAZPACHO

Yield: 12 servings
Serving Size: 2/3 cup

Ingredients
4 cups V-8 juice
1 Tbsp. lemon juice
1 cup cucumber, thinly sliced
1/2 green pepper, chopped
2 cups tomatoes, peeled, seeded, and chopped
1/2 cup red onion, chopped
1/4 cup green onion, sliced
Hot pepper sauce to taste

Method
1. To peel and seed tomatoes, bring a small pan of water to a boil. Put in 1 whole fresh tomato so that water covers the entire tomato. Leave in water 30 to 45 seconds. Remove tomato and immediately run under cold water. Pierce skin with a sharp knife and peel. Cut in half and squeeze gently to remove seeds.
2. Set aside 1/4 to 1/2 of the raw chopped and sliced vegetables to garnish the soup. Add the remaining vegetables to the juice and refrigerate 2 hours. If soup is chunkier than desired, it can be blended slightly.
3. Serve cold with abundant garnishes.

MIXED-FIBER PILAF

Yield: 10 servings
Serving Size: 1/3 cup

Ingredients
1/3 cup bulgur wheat
1/2 cup quick brown rice
1/4 quick barley
1/2 cup onion, chopped
1/2 cup mushrooms, thinly sliced
2 tsp. olive oil
1 1/2 cups chicken broth or water
1/8 tsp. thyme
Pepper to taste

Method
1. Heat olive oil in a large skillet and saute onions and mushrooms until onions are translucent and all liquid is evaporated.
2. Add bulgur, rice, and barley and continue to saute until lightly golden brown.
3. Add chicken broth and simmer covered on low for 15 minutes or until grains are tender and liquid has been absorbed.

INDEX TO RECIPES

This index lists items by the menu in which they appear. B = breakfast, L = lunch, and D = dinner. For example, the entry Sugarless Blueberry Muffins, B19, indicates that the recipe is found in breakfast 19.

Page numbers refer to the Snack or Picnics & Barbecues sections of *Month of Meals 3*.

Now That We've Tickled Your Taste Buds, Dig Into Our Recipe-Packed Pantry of Cookbooks and Menu Planners

Month of Meals

A "Special Occasion" section offers tips for brunches, holidays, parties, and restaurants to give you delicious dining options in most any setting. Oven Fried Fish, Sloppy Joes, Crab Cakes, many others. 57 pages. Spiral-bound. #CMPMOM
Member: $9.95
Nonmember: $12.50

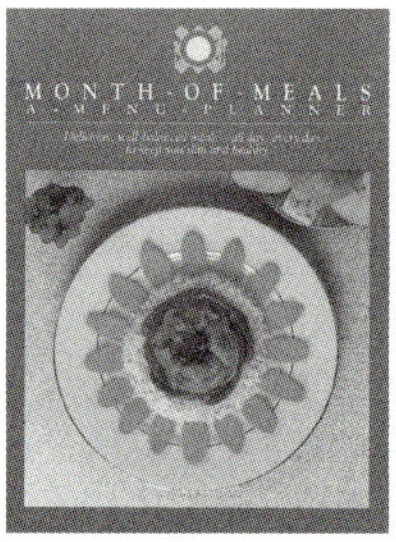

Month of Meals 2

Tips and meal suggestions for Mexican, Italian, and Chinese restaurants are featured. Quick-to-fix and ethnic recipes are also included. Veal Piccata, Beef Burritos, Chop Suey, and more. 64 pages. Spiral-bound. #CMPMOM2
Member: $9.95
Nonmember: $12.50

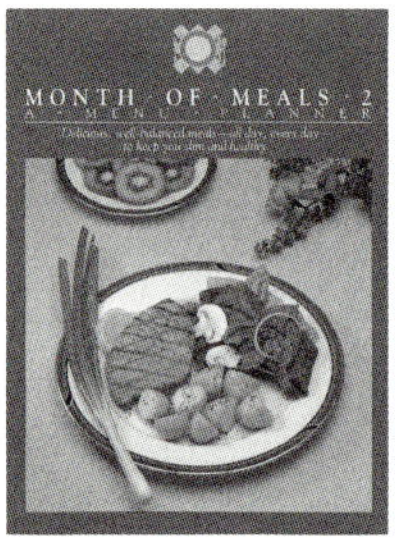

Month of Meals 3

Special sections offer valuable tips: reading ingredient labels on packages; preparing meals for picnics and barbeques; planning meals when you're ill. Kentucky Fried Chicken, Stouffer's Macaroni and Cheese, many others. 72 pages. Spiral-bound. #CMPMOM3
Member: $9.95
Nonmember: $12.50

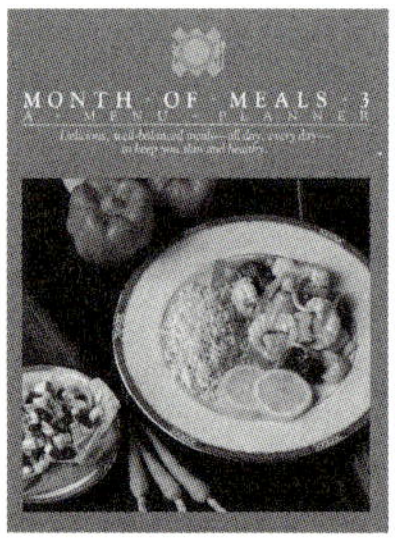

Month of Meals 4

Hints for turning family-size meals into "planned overs" keep left-overs from going to waste. Meal plans for one or two people are featured. Oven Crispy Chicken, Beef Stroganoff, Meatloaf, Pot Roast, many others. 74 pages. Spiral-bound. #CMPMOM4
Member: $9.95
Nonmember: $12.50

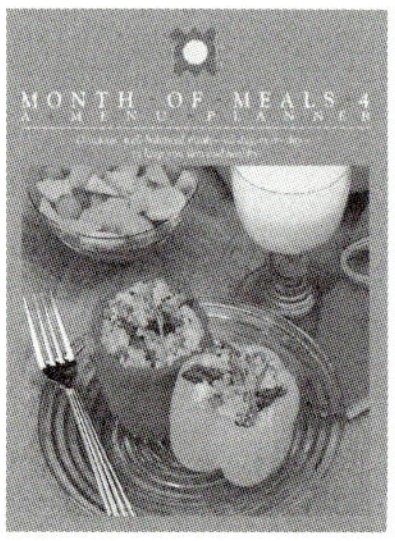

NEW!
Coming in June, 1994
Month of Meals 5

A month's worth of fresh new meal plans with a special focus on vegetarian selections. #CMPMOM5
Member: $9.95 **Nonmember: $12.50**

SAVE 10%! Month of Meals Sets

Set of *Month of Meals* volumes 1-3. #CMPSET3
Member: $26.85
Nonmember: $33.75

Set of *Month of Meals* volumes 1-4. #CMPSET4
Member: $35.80
Nonmember: $45.00

Healthy HomeStyle Cookbook

Come and get it! Here's home cooking at its best--and healthiest. More than 150 recipes low in fat, cholesterol, sugar, and calories. Try Dutch Apple Pancakes, Sweet and Sour Meatballs, Chicken Nuggets, many others. Includes energy- and time-saving tips for microwaving and freezing. "Lay-flat" binding allows hands-free reference to any recipe. 192 pages. Softcover. #CCBHHS
Member: $9.95 **Nonmember: $12.50**

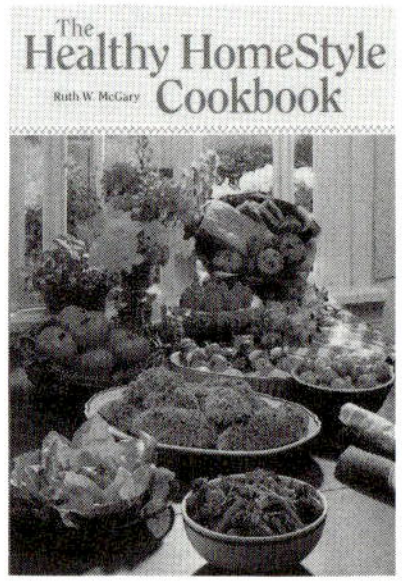

Holiday Cookbook

From Eggnog to Cranberry Rolls, our *Holiday Cookbook* will fill your table with tempting recipes from traditional Thanksgiving, Christmas, and Hannukah feasts to savory meal for any occasion. 219 pages. Hardcover. #CCBH
Member: $17.95
Nonmember: $19.95

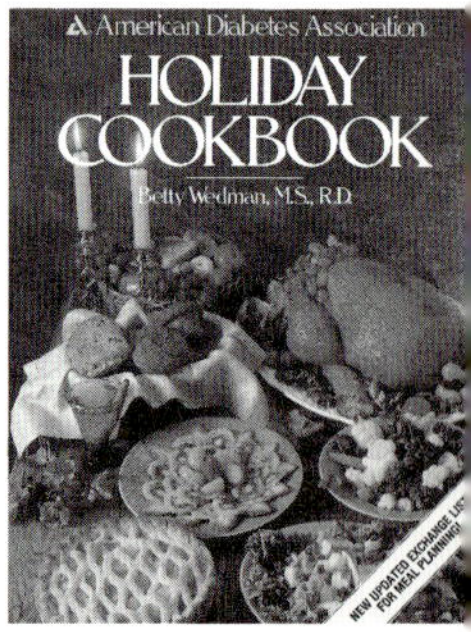

Special Celebrations and Parties Cookbook

Cheesecake? Brownies? On MY diet? Yes! Whether it's a Fourth of July barbecue, Mother's Day brunch, or birthday bash, these recipes will tempt everyone's taste buds. 256 pages. Hardcover. #CCBSCP
Member: $17.95
Nomember: $19.95

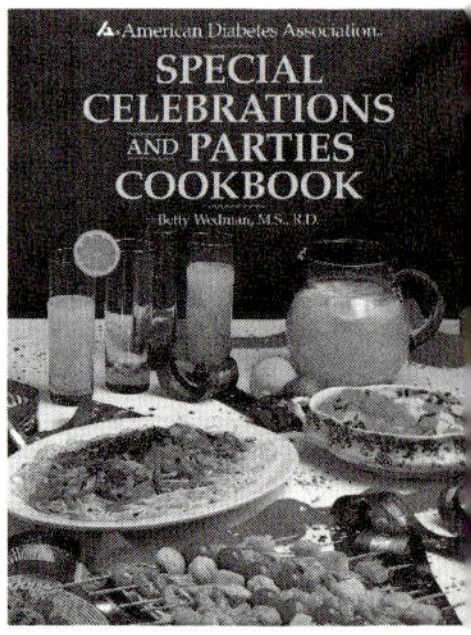

SAVE 10%! Holiday Celebration Set

Includes *Holiday Cookbook* and *Special Celebrations & Parties Cookbook.*
#CCBSET2
Member: $32.90 **Nonmember: $35.90**

Yes! Please send me the following:

____ copies of *Month of Meals* .... $ ______
____ copies of *Month of Meals 2* .... $ ______
____ copies of *Month of Meals 3* .... $ ______
____ copies of *Month of Meals 4* .... $ ______
____ copies of *Month of Meals Set of 3* .... $ ______
____ copies of *Month of Meals Set of 4* .... $ ______
____ copies of *Healthy HomeStyle* .... $ ______
____ copies of *Holiday Cookbook* .... $ ______
____ copies of *Special Celebrations Cookbook* .... $ ______
____ copies of *Holiday Celebrations Set* .... $ ______
Publications Subtotal .... $ ______
Virginia residents add 4.5% state sales tax .... $ ______
Add shipping & handling (see chart) .... $ ______
Add $15 for each international shipment .... $ ______
GRAND TOTAL .... $ ______

Allow 2-3 weeks for shipment. There's an extra $3 charge for each additional shipping address. Prices are subject to change without notice. Foreign orders must be paid in U.S. funds, drawn on a U.S. bank.

______
Name
______
Address
______
City/State/Zip

____ Payment enclosed (check or money order)
Charge my: ☐ MasterCard ☐ VISA ☐ Amex
Account Number ______
Signature ______ Exp. Date ______

CH39401

Shipping & Handling Chart

Up to $30.00.......	add $3.00
$30.01-$50.00......	add $4.00
Above $50.00......	add 8% of order

Mail to:
American Diabetes Association
1970 Chain Bridge Road
McLean, VA 22109-0592

Yes! Please send me the following:

____ copies of *Month of Meals* .... $ ______
____ copies of *Month of Meals 2* .... $ ______
____ copies of *Month of Meals 3* .... $ ______
____ copies of *Month of Meals 4* .... $ ______
____ copies of *Month of Meals Set of 3* .... $ ______
____ copies of *Month of Meals Set of 4* .... $ ______
____ copies of *Healthy HomeStyle* .... $ ______
____ copies of *Holiday Cookbook* .... $ ______
____ copies of *Special Celebrations Cookbook* .... $ ______
____ copies of *Holiday Celebrations Set* .... $ ______
Publications Subtotal .... $ ______
Virginia residents add 4.5% state sales tax .... $ ______
Add shipping & handling (see chart) .... $ ______
Add $15 for each international shipment .... $ ______
GRAND TOTAL .... $ ______

Allow 2-3 weeks for shipment. There's an extra $3 charge for each additional shipping address. Prices are subject to change without notice. Foreign orders must be paid in U.S. funds, drawn on a U.S. bank.

______
Name
______
Address
______
City/State/Zip

____ Payment enclosed (check or money order)
Charge my: ☐ MasterCard ☐ VISA ☐ Amex
Account Number ______
Signature ______ Exp. Date ______

CH39401

Shipping & Handling Chart

Up to $30.00.......	add $3.00
$30.01-$50.00.....	add $4.00
Above $50.00......	add 8% of order

Mail to:
American Diabetes Association
1970 Chain Bridge Road
McLean, VA 22109-0592

Yes! Please send me the following:

____ copies of *Month of Meals* .... $ ______
____ copies of *Month of Meals 2* .... $ ______
____ copies of *Month of Meals 3* .... $ ______
____ copies of *Month of Meals 4* .... $ ______
____ copies of *Month of Meals Set of 3* .... $ ______
____ copies of *Month of Meals Set of 4* .... $ ______
____ copies of *Healthy HomeStyle* .... $ ______
____ copies of *Holiday Cookbook* .... $ ______
____ copies of *Special Celebrations Cookbook* .... $ ______
____ copies of *Holiday Celebrations Set* .... $ ______
Publications Subtotal .... $ ______
Virginia residents add 4.5% state sales tax .... $ ______
Add shipping & handling (see chart) .... $ ______
Add $15 for each international shipment .... $ ______
GRAND TOTAL .... $ ______

Allow 2-3 weeks for shipment. There's an extra $3 charge for each additional shipping address. Prices are subject to change without notice. Foreign orders must be paid in U.S. funds, drawn on a U.S. bank.

______
Name
______
Address
______
City/State/Zip

____ Payment enclosed (check or money order)
Charge my: ☐ MasterCard ☐ VISA ☐ Amex
Account Number ______
Signature ______ Exp. Date ______

CH39401

Shipping & Handling Chart

Up to $30.00.......	add $3.00
$30.01-$50.00......	add $4.00
Above $50.00......	add 8% of order

Mail to:
American Diabetes Association
1970 Chain Bridge Road
McLean, VA 22109-0592

Order TOLL FREE!
1-800-232-3472
(Monday through Friday, 9:00 a.m. - 5 p.m. Eastern Time)
VISA, MasterCard, American Express accepted.

Our catalog is FREE. Just give us a call and we'll send you a copy.

Order TOLL FREE!
1-800-232-3472
(Monday through Friday, 9:00 a.m. - 5 p.m. Eastern Time)
VISA, MasterCard, American Express accepted.

Our catalog is FREE. Just give us a call and we'll send you a copy.

Order TOLL FREE!
1-800-232-3472
(Monday through Friday, 9:00 a.m. - 5 p.m. Eastern Time)
VISA, MasterCard, American Express accepted.

Our catalog is FREE. Just give us a call and we'll send you a copy.